# Discussion on TCM Basics Through Understanding of

# the Yellow Emperor's Inner Canon

## By Yingxiong Feng

DISCUSSION ON TCM BASICS THROUGH UNDERSTANDING OF THE YELLOW EMPEROR'S INNER CANON

**First edition. March 11, 2024.**

Copyright © 2024 yingxiong feng.

ISBN: 979-8224706495

Written by yingxiong feng.

# Table of Contents

# Introduction

The Huangdi Neijing, also known as the Yellow Emperor's Inner Canon, is one of the classical works of ancient Chinese medicine and is considered the foundation of traditional Chinese medicine (TCM). It is attributed to the Yellow Emperor, but in reality, it is a compilation of the medical experiences of various masters from different periods.

The Huangdi Neijing consists of two parts: Suwen (Basic Questions) and Ling Shu (Spiritual Pivot). Suwen primarily discusses fundamental medical theories, including concepts such as yin and yang, the five elements, qi, blood, and bodily fluids, as well as the system of organs, meridians, and collaterals. On the other hand, Ling Shu focuses on details such as meridians, acupuncture points, and the functions of organs. Together, these two parts form the theoretical framework of TCM.

In summary, Suwen, through exploration of topics like yin and yang, the five elements, qi, blood, bodily fluids, organs, meridians, etiology, pathogenesis, and treatment methods, establishes the fundamental theoretical system of TCM. This classic work emphasizes a holistic perspective, highlighting the importance of balance and harmony. It introduces many unique medical concepts, laying a solid foundation for the development of traditional Chinese medicine.

In practical application, the theories presented in the "Suwen" provide Chinese medicine practitioners with a rich framework for contemplation and treatment methods.

The "Suwen" is divided into 81 sections, covering a wide range of fields including medicine, philosophy, and natural sciences. The main contents of the "Suwen" include Yin and Yang, Five Elements, Qi, Blood, Bodily Fluids, Organs, Meridians, Etiology and Pathogenesis, Treatment Methods and Acupuncture, Prevention and Health Maintenance.

The "Suwen" initially discusses the theories of yin and yang and the five elements, emphasizing the laws of change in the universe and the human body. Yin and yang, along with the five elements, are core concepts in ancient Chinese philosophy and are integral to the overall theoretical framework of traditional Chinese medicine.

The "Suwen" clarifies the concepts of qi, blood, and bodily fluids, highlighting the importance of their balance for human health. The flow and abundance of qi, blood, and bodily fluids are closely related to the well-being of the human body.

The text elaborately discusses the concepts of organs and meridians, revealing the physiological functions and interrelationships of each organ. The theory of organs and meridians forms the foundation for the diagnosis and treatment in Chinese medicine, allowing practitioners to assess the health status of the body by observing changes in the organs.

The "Suwen" extensively explores the causes and developmental processes of diseases, introducing the concepts of etiology and pathogenesis. It emphasizes the impact of external factors, internal imbalances, emotional factors, etc., on the occurrence of diseases, laying the foundation for later differentiation of syndromes.

The "Suwen" systematically summarizes various treatment methods, including pharmacotherapy, acupuncture, dietary regulation, and more. Particularly, the "Lingshu" section delves deeper into the principles and applications of acupuncture.

The text introduces the concept of "treating before illness occurs" and underscores the importance of prevention and health maintenance. By adjusting diet, lifestyle, and other factors, potential health issues can be preemptively addressed before the onset of diseases.

In Western society, there has been a gradual rise in the translation and study of the Huangdi Neijing, making it one of the representatives of traditional Chinese medicine internationally. Western scholars have conducted in-depth research on it, attempting to engage in dialogue and integration of its theories with Western medicine. The Huangdi Neijing has exerted a certain influence on Western medicine, particularly in the fields of integrative medicine and traditional Chinese medical treatment methods. Some Western medical researchers have incorporated certain concepts into their studies, facilitating communication and collaboration between different medical systems.

However, it is essential to note that due to fundamental differences between Chinese and Western medical systems, the Huangdi Neijing has not been as widely applied in clinical practice in Western society as it has in China. In the West, the understanding of TCM theories is still evolving, and there are ongoing debates and controversies in this regard.

# Chapter 1

# Theoretical System Of Traditional Chinese Medicine

Traditional Chinese Medicine (TCM) is a traditional medical science that explores the physiology, pathology, diagnosis, prevention, and treatment of diseases, as well as health preservation and rehabilitation of the human body. It possesses a distinctive theoretical framework.

Originating in ancient China, TCM's theoretical system took shape during the Warring States to the Qin and Han periods. The theoretical foundation of TCM is built upon ancient Chinese philosophical ideas and traditional culture. It has evolved through the accumulation of extensive healthcare experiences and theoretical summaries over an extended period.

The foundational theory of Traditional Chinese Medicine is a theoretical summary of the laws governing human life activities and disease changes. The milestone in the formation of the TCM theoretical system is marked by the emergence of the Huangdi Neijing (Yellow Emperor's Inner Canon).

The Huangdi Neijing assimilated significant achievements from various disciplines such as astronomy, calendrics, meteorology, mathematics, biology, and geography prior to the Qin and Han dynasties. Guided by the principles of the unity of Qi and the Yin-Yang Five Elements theory, it synthesized medical accomplishments and treatment experiences before the Spring and Autumn and Warring

States periods. The Huangdi Neijing established the theoretical principles of TCM, systematically expounding on issues related to physiology, pathology, meridians, anatomy, diagnosis, treatment, prevention, and more. It laid the foundation for the development of TCM and served as the theoretical source.

The Huangdi Neijing, along with Treatise on Cold Damage and Miscellaneous Diseases by Zhang Zhongjing from the Han dynasty, respectively, form the foundational works of basic TCM theory and the principles of syndrome differentiation and treatment. Together with the Shennong Bencao Jing (Divine Farmer's Materia Medica) and the Nan Jing (Classic of Difficult Issues), these texts have been revered by generations of medical practitioners as the Four Classics, exerting a profound influence on the subsequent development of medicine.

Since the Tang and Song dynasties, through the Ming and Qing dynasties, many medical practitioners, building upon the achievements of their predecessors, boldly innovated and proposed unique insights based on their own practical experiences. This led to new breakthroughs and developments in the academic field of Traditional Chinese Medicine. Each generation of medical practitioners had distinctive characteristics in their medical practices, contributing innovative ideas from different perspectives, enriching and advancing TCM, and promoting the development of both theoretical and clinical aspects of TCM.

The study of TCM theory has become a global research topic, with scholars from various countries making significant contributions. The diagnostic and treatment methods of TCM have been widely accepted by the public in mainstream countries such as the United States.

## The fundamental content of the theoretical framework in TCM

Traditional Chinese Medicine has absorbed philosophical achievements from before the Han dynasty, applying important philosophical concepts and theories such as Qi, Yin-Yang, the Five

Elements, form and spirit, and the relationship between heaven and humans to explain medical issues, making them important concepts and theories within TCM.

TCM uses the theory of the Five Elements—wood, fire, earth, metal, and water—to argue for the organic connections between different parts of the human body, as well as the unity between humans and their environment, illustrating that the human body is a microcosm.

The theories of Zangxiang (Organ Manifestations), Meridians, and the dynamics of Qi, Blood, Essence, and Fluids are aspects of Traditional Chinese Medicine that pertain to the understanding of normal physiological phenomena. Among these, the Zangxiang theory is considered the core of the TCM theoretical framework.

Zangxiang theory investigates the regularities of organ activities and their interrelationships within the human body. It posits that the human body centers around five Zang organs—Heart, Liver, Spleen, Lung, and Kidney—coordinated with six Fu organs—Gallbladder, Stomach, Small Intestine, Large Intestine, Bladder, and Triple Burner. These are supported by Qi, Blood, Essence, and Fluids as the material foundation. Through the meridians, these elements connect the internal organs with the external sensory organs, limbs, and the entire body, forming an organic whole. This interconnected system is unified with the external environment.

The theory of Qi, Blood, Essence, and Fluids primarily explores the material composition of life and the material foundation of life activities.

Meridian theory is the study of the composition, course, distribution, physiological functions, pathological changes of the human meridian system, and it serves as a theoretical guide for clinical treatment. Meridians are the pathways through which Qi and Blood circulate in the body, crisscrossing and interconnecting to form a network that links the internal and external aspects of the body, as well as the organs, limbs, and joints, creating an organic whole.

Traditional Chinese Medicine believes that the occurrence of diseases results from pathogenic factors affecting the human body, disrupting normal physiological activities and causing imbalances in the organs, meridians, Yin-Yang, and Qi-Blood. The etiology of diseases can be categorized into six external pathogenic factors (Wind, Cold, Summer Heat, Dampness, Dryness, Fire), epidemic factors, seven emotions (Joy, Anger, Worry, Thought, Grief, Fear, Surprise), inappropriate diet, improper balance between exertion and rest, external injuries, and prenatal influences.

Establishing the concept of etiology based on symptoms, signs, and syndromes is a distinctive criterion and major characteristic in confirming the causes of diseases in TCM.

The mechanism of pathological changes, abbreviated as pathomechanism or pathology, is the theory that explores the regularities of pathological changes in the human body. It encompasses general principles of pathologic changes such as the dominance or decline of pathogenic and righteous factors, imbalances in Yin and Yang, disturbances in Qi, Blood, and Essence, abnormalities in Fluids, as well as irregularities in the organs, meridians, and other physiological aspects.

Diagnosis and pattern differentiation in Traditional Chinese Medicine involve four methods of examining diseases, commonly known as the Four Diagnoses: inspection (looking), listening and smelling (hearing), questioning (inquiring), and palpation (touching).

Inspection involves purposefully observing the patient's spirit, appearance, facial features, sensory organs, tongue condition, and excretions to understand the illness and detect organ dysfunction.

Listening and smelling entail distinguishing the inherent condition of the disease by paying attention to the patient's language, breathing sounds, and odors emitted from the patient's body.

Questioning involves inquiries directed to the patient and those familiar with the patient, aiming to understand the patient's usual health status, the cause of the illness, the progression of symptoms, and the patient's self-awareness of their condition.

Palpation includes examining the patient's pulse and other parts of the body to assess internal changes. Among the Four Diagnoses, key aspects include observing the spirit, facial color, tongue condition, inquiring about symptoms, and examining the pulse.

Each of the Four Diagnoses has specific examination content that cannot be substituted for others. It is necessary to combine all four for a systematic and comprehensive acquisition of clinical data, providing a reliable basis for pattern differentiation.

Adopting proactive preventive or therapeutic measures to prevent the occurrence and development of diseases, known as "treating before illness," is a fundamental principle in the field of Traditional Chinese Medicine.

The study of TCM health preservation explores the regularities of human life, elucidates theories and methods for enhancing constitution, preventing diseases, and prolonging life. It regards essence, Qi, and spirit as the three treasures of the human body, emphasizing that the way of health preservation must adhere to the principles of Yin-Yang, harmonize with numerical techniques, nurture both form and spirit, balance Yin and Yang, be cautious in daily activities, coordinate the functions of organs, adapt to appropriate levels of activity, preserve Qi, and consolidate essence. Health preservation represents the most proactive preventive measures.

Seeking the root cause of illness, understanding the regular and adapting to changes, guiding treatment based on the situation, and pursuing balance represent the fundamental concepts in the treatment of diseases in Traditional Chinese Medicine. The basic principles of TCM treatment include rectifying the primary cause, addressing symptoms and root causes, regulating Yin and Yang, harmonizing Qi and Blood, adjusting the functions of organs, considering both the physical and mental aspects, integrating the diagnosis and syndrome, and tailoring treatment based on individual differences.

Prevention, treatment, and rehabilitation are three distinct yet interconnected theories and methods within TCM for combating diseases. These principles play a crucial role in clinical medical practice and contribute significantly to ensuring people's health and longevity.

Emphasizing the unity of humanity and nature, and the interconnectedness of all things, is one of the fundamental characteristics of Traditional Chinese Medicine. The human body is considered an organic whole, composed of various organs and systems that are inseparable and interrelated. Each organ is a component of the body's holistic system and cannot exist independently outside this totality. Qi, blood, essence, body fluids, and liquid are the basic substances that constitute the human body and sustain its vital activities. In other words, Qi, blood, essence, fluids, and liquids are all derived from a singular Qi.

Humans and nature are unified, sharing common laws and are both subject to the governing movements of Yin and Yang and the Five Elements. Moreover, there are specific correlating relationships in many of their respective movement laws. Human physiological activities change in accordance with the movements of the natural world and the variations in natural conditions.

The climate exhibits rhythmic changes throughout the four seasons, presenting as spring warmth, summer heat, autumn dryness, and winter cold. Consequently, the human body undergoes adaptive changes in response to these seasonal variations. In hot weather, the circulation of Qi and blood accelerates, pores open up, and sweating is profuse. In cold weather, the circulation of Qi and blood slows down, pores contract, and sweating is limited. This clearly illustrates the impact of seasonal climate changes on the physiological functions of the human body.

The movement of Qi and blood in the human body not only varies with the changing seasons but also follows a rhythmic pattern in response to the alternation of day and night. For instance, the Yang Qi in the human body exhibits regular fluctuations with the onset of morning, reaching its peak at noon, weakening in the evening, and declining around midnight.

Traditional Chinese Medicine places significant emphasis on the impact of geographical regions on the human body. Growth differs between the north and the south, terrains vary in elevation, constitutions are categorized by Yin and Yang, diets vary from rich to simple, and there are differences in climate from cold to warm, all of which contribute to variations in disease manifestations.

Humans live within social environments, and changes in social ecology are closely related to mental and physical health, as well as the occurrence of diseases. Differences in social roles and status, along with changes in the social environment, not only affect people's mental and physical functions but also result in different disease patterns.

TCM starts from the holistic concept of the unity of heaven, earth, and humanity, emphasizing that medical research should have knowledge of astronomy above, geography below, and human affairs in between. It advocates for treating diseases without losing compassion, believing that "one who does not understand heaven, earth, and humanity cannot be a physician."

The discipline of TCM treatment emphasizes the need to tailor the treatment to the individual, taking into account the timing, location, and specific characteristics of the patient. It advocates starting from a holistic perspective, comprehensively understanding and analyzing the condition. Attention should not only be given to the local manifestations of the disease and the pathological changes in the affected organs but also to the relationships between the affected organs and other organs.

The focus is on grasping the overall imbalance of Yin-Yang and Qi-Blood, working towards harmonizing the overall balance of Yin-Yang, Qi-Blood, and organ functions. The approach involves supporting the correct (healthy) factors, expelling the pathogenic (disease-causing) factors, eliminating the systemic impact of the disease, and breaking the chain of pathological reactions caused by the disease between different organs.

By addressing the overall imbalances and applying treatments that harmonize the entire system, TCM aims to eliminate the pathogenic factors and achieve the goal of curing the disease.

"Differentiation of Syndromes For Treatment" refers to the combined principles of syndrome differentiation and treatment, serving as both the fundamental principle for understanding and treating diseases in Traditional Chinese Medicine and the basic method for diagnosing and preventing diseases. It is also one of the fundamental characteristics of the TCM theoretical system.

The occurrence and development of any disease are always manifested through specific symptoms, signs, and other disease phenomena. People typically reveal the essence of a disease by observing these disease manifestations.

Symptoms represent the individual surface phenomena of a disease, indicating abnormal sensations or pathological changes subjectively felt by the patient. Examples include headaches, fever, cough, nausea, vomiting, and so on. Symptoms are essential for understanding the nature of a disease.

Differentiation of syndromes, a unique concept in Traditional Chinese Medicine, is the core of understanding and treating diseases in TCM. A syndrome is composed of symptoms, but it is not a simple summation of various symptoms. Instead, it captures the essential meaning of symptoms through phenomena, clarifies their internal connections, and thereby reveals the essence of the disease.

Disease is manifested through syndromes, reflecting the entire process of pathological changes and the basic laws of occurrence, development, and transformation.

Common methods of syndrome differentiation used in clinical practice include Eight Principles differentiation, Zang-Fu organ differentiation, Qi-Blood-Fluid differentiation, Six Channels differentiation, Defensive Qi-Vital Energy Qi- Nutritious Qi -Blood differentiation, Triple Burner differentiation, and etiological differentiation. While these methods each have their distinct characteristics and focus on different aspects of diagnosing various diseases, they are interconnected and complement each other.

Guided by the holistic perspective, a meticulous clinical observation is conducted using the Four Diagnoses. This involves examining a series of symptoms and signs manifested by the patient under the influence of pathogenic factors. Based on the principle of "differential diagnosis to seek the cause," reasoning is applied to determine the etiology of the illness. Combining geographical environment, seasonal factors, climate, as well as the patient's constitution, gender, occupation, and other specific factors, a detailed analysis is performed to uncover the essence of the disease. This process leads to a conclusive syndrome differentiation, allowing for the determination of treatment principles. Finally, a suitable prescription of herbal medicine or therapeutic approach is chosen for treatment. This constitutes the fundamental process of clinical syndrome differentiation and treatment in Traditional Chinese Medicine.

In the practice of syndrome differentiation and treatment, it is crucial to understand the relationship between the disease and the syndrome. One must distinguish not only the disease but also the syndrome, with a greater emphasis on differentiating the syndrome. The syndrome reflects the various stages and pathological changes of the disease. Therefore, as the disease progresses, different syndromes may appear, and treatment should be tailored according to the specific syndromes that manifest during the course of the illness.

In the same disease, different syndromes may occur, and in different diseases, similar syndromes may manifest. For example, in cases of jaundice, some may exhibit symptoms of damp-heat syndrome, requiring treatment to clear heat and promote dampness elimination. Others may show signs of cold-damp syndrome, necessitating treatment to warm and dispel cold-dampness. This phenomenon is known as treating the same disease with different approaches.

Similarly, different diseases, during their progression, may develop similar syndromes. Therefore, they can be treated using the same method. For instance, if two distinct diseases exhibit similar syndromes, they can both be treated with a common therapeutic approach. This is referred to as treating different diseases with the same method.

# Chapter 2

## Understanding The Essential Philosophy Of Qi As The Vital Energy

Traditional Chinese Medicine believes that the universe and all things originally stem from a single vital force, which is categorized into Yin and Yang when differentiated. Further division within the Yin and Yang leads to the concept of the Five Elements.

There exists a tangible and intangible entity in the universe, referred to as "qi" in ancient Chinese philosophy. Qi is an extremely refined and subtle substance beyond the perception of the naked eye.

In Chinese ancient philosophy, Qi is the fundamental category that signifies the existence of material. It is a dynamic and supremely refined material entity, constituting the most basic element of the universe's myriad phenomena.

In the theoretical framework of traditional Chinese medicine regarding the vital substance system, including Qi, blood, essence, bodily fluids, and secretions, Qi is considered the foundational element for the structure of the human body and the maintenance of life activities. It is a highly vigorous, incessantly moving, and extremely subtle substance, representing the unity of vital substances and physiological functions. Among the various specific material concepts within the vital substance system, Qi is the most encompassing concept.

The "Huangdi Neijing" describes the universe as "Tai Xu", a vast and boundless empty space filled with inexhaustible primordial Qi possessing vitalizing capabilities. This primordial Qi permeates the expanse of the universe, governs the earth, and initiates celestial and terrestrial processes. All tangible forms owe their existence to the vitalizing power of primordial Qi. Primordial Qi serves as the foundation of the universe, the origin and destination of all things in the world. Qi is the fundamental substance that constitutes the universe, originally unified but divided into Yin and Yang. Qi represents the contradictory unity of Yin and Yang.

Clear Yang forms the heavens, while turbid Yin forms the earth. Earthly Qi rises as clouds, and celestial Qi descends as rain. Rain originates from the Qi of the earth, and clouds arise from the Qi of the heavens. "Heavenly Qi" is the clear Yang energy in the natural world, and "Earthly Qi" is the turbid Yin energy in the natural world. Yin Qi is heavy and descends to condense into tangible objects, creating the colorful landscape of the earth. Yang Qi is clear and light, ascending and dispersing into the formless Tai Xu, shaping the vast expanse of the heavens.

The interaction of the ascending and descending Yin and Yang Qi in the heavens and earth influences and shapes everything in the universe.

Traditional Chinese medicine starts from the fundamental viewpoint that Qi is the origin of the universe and the essential element that constitutes everything under heaven and earth. It believes that Qi is also the origin of life and the basic material that forms life. At the beginning of human existence, there is first the transformation of Qi, followed by the formation of physical shape. The human body is an organism constantly undergoing the transformative actions of Qi, including rising, falling, exiting, and entering. The growth, aging, health, and disease of a person all stem from Qi. The life and death of a person entirely depend on Qi. Life begins when Qi gathers, health is maintained when Qi is strong, weakness ensues when Qi declines, and death occurs when Qi disperses.

Blood, essence, body fluids, and other vital substances are also fundamental to life, but they are all generated from Qi. Qi is the most basic material that constitutes the human body and maintains its vital activities.

The human form is composed of Qi, and the mental consciousness and thought activities of humans are also a manifestation of the Qi generated by the material body.

The contrasting unity and movement of Yin and Yang in Qi are demonstrated through interactions such as ascending and descending, exiting and entering, movement and stillness, gathering and dispersing, clarity and turbidity in the heavens and earth. These are specific manifestations of the movement of Qi.

Qi is the material foundation of the universe, forming into shape when gathered and dispersing into Qi when scattered. In the life of the human body, Qi gives rise to form, and form returns to Qi. When Qi accumulates, form emerges; when Qi disperses, form perishes. The existence of human life entirely depends on this Qi.

When Yang is in motion and scatters, it transforms into Qi, and when Yin is still and condenses, it takes on a specific form. The mutual interaction of Yin and Yang in motion and stillness is the fundamental reason for the opposing directional processes of Qi transforming into form and form dissolving into Qi.

Metabolism is a fundamental characteristic of life. The life and death of a person depend on Qi, which serves as the material foundation for sustaining life activities. In the "Su Wen," it is stated: "Taste returns to form, form returns to Qi, Qi returns to essence, essence returns to transformation. Essence consumes Qi, form consumes taste, transformation generates essence, and Qi generates form." The perpetual movement of Qi and transformation is inherent in the entire process of life, and without this metabolic process, there would be no life.

For the proper functioning of the organs and their ascending and descending movements, as well as orderly exits and entrances, it is crucial to maintain the normal physiological activities described as "clear Yang exiting the upper orifices, turbid Yin exiting the lower orifices; clear Yang spreading through the skin, turbid Yin circulating through the five viscera; clear Yang filling the four limbs, turbid Yin returning to the six bowels." This ensures the continuous metabolism between the organism and the external environment, guaranteeing the constant self-renewal of the material foundation of life – Qi.

All organs and entrails rely on Qi for their function. Qi values harmony and prefers to flow and spread like water. All diseases, whether external or internal, deficient or excessive, acute or chronic, arise from Qi, hence the saying "all diseases are born of Qi" or the malfunctioning of Qi. Whether a disease is characterized by deficiency or excess, cold or heat, or any other pathological change that cannot be named, seeking its root cause can always be attributed to Qi alone. The location of Qi imbalance is the root of the disease. The occurrence and development of all diseases are related to the abnormal generation and flow of Qi.

In Traditional Chinese Medicine diagnostics, by examining the manifestations of diseases in the five organs, one can determine the deficiency or sufficiency of vital Qi. The rise and fall of the righteous Qi can be observed through complexion, physical appearance, voice, mental state, and pulse among other aspects, with mental state and pulse being particularly important. The presence or absence of the mental spirit is a sign of life activities, with the spirit relying on essence and Qi as its material foundation, reflecting the prosperity or decline of organ Qi and blood. If the primal Qi is slightly deficient, the spirit slightly fades; if the primal Qi is greatly deficient, the spirit completely vanishes. By observing the complexion, one can also discern the prosperity or decline of the internal organs, the deficiency or sufficiency of Qi and blood, and the depth of pathogenic Qi.

The flow of pulse Qi travels through the meridians, and the abundance or decline of Qi can be reflected in pulse diagnosis, with the Qi ultimately returning to the lungs. In diagnosis, examining the state of stomach Qi is crucial in determining the course of disease, whether it will progress favorably or unfavorably, or lead to life or death. Life is sustained with stomach Qi, and without it, death occurs.

The fundamental principle of treatment lies in supporting the righteous and expelling the pathogenic. Expelling pathogenic factors is done to support the righteous, and supporting the righteous is done to expel the pathogenic. The goal of treatment is to regulate the blood and Qi, promoting harmony. When Qi is in harmony, it is righteous; when harmony is lost, it becomes pathogenic. The key to treating Qi is to achieve harmony, not only by using Qi-regulating herbs to smooth the flow of Qi but also by adjusting the imbalance of Yin and Yang in the organs through various therapeutic methods. This aims to restore the dynamic balance of Yin and Yang, Qi, and blood circulation within the body.

Within the Yin and Yang dynamics in the human body, there is an emphasis on the primacy of Yang, asserting that when Yang Qi is strong, Yin Qi naturally follows. Yang Qi is considered Yang, and Yin Qi is regarded as Yin.

Under certain conditions, mutual transformation can occur between Yin and Yang. Yin can transform into Yang, and Yang can also transform into Yin. For example, in the transformation of cold and heat syndromes, the nature of the pathological cold or heat changes, leading to a corresponding alteration in their Yin-Yang attributes. In the process of the body's Qi movement, material substances are associated with Yin, while physiological functions are associated with Yang.

Traditional Chinese medicine uses the symbols of water and fire to represent Yin and Yang, with water representing Yin and fire representing Yang. This reflects the fundamental characteristics of Yin and Yang, such as water being cold and descending, and fire being hot and rising.

Yin and Yang are inherent attributes of Qi. The movement of Qi involves the opposing and unified dynamics of Yin and Yang. Within the Qi of the human body, it can be categorized into Yin and Yang based on their characteristics. The Qi that possesses a warming and propelling function in the human body is referred to as Yang Qi, while the Qi that plays a role in nourishing and moistening is called Yin Qi.

In terms of physiological activities in the human body, the generation of various functional activities (Yang) inevitably involves the consumption of certain nutritional substances (Yin), leading to the process known as "Yang grows, Yin diminishes." Conversely, the transformation of various nutritional substances (Yin) also necessitates the consumption of a certain amount of energy (Yang).

The absence of Yin when there is Yang is referred to as "solitary Yang," and the absence of Yang when there is Yin is referred to as "solitary Yin." Without Yin, Yang cannot generate, and without Yang, Yin cannot thrive. In such a scenario, all living beings would cease to exist, unable to undergo vital processes and growth. In the course of life activities, if the normal interdependence of Yin and Yang is disrupted, it can lead to the onset of diseases and even pose a threat to life.

For instance, in patients with prolonged loss of appetite, it often manifests as weakness in spleen Qi (Yang). Since the spleen and stomach are considered the foundation of acquired factors and the source of Qi and blood transformation, a weakness in spleen Qi (Yang) results in insufficient transformation, leading to Yin (blood) deficiency. This can be described as a condition of both Yang deficiency and Yin deficiency in Qi and blood.

In the progression of a disease, the transformation of Yin and Yang often manifests under certain conditions, including the transformation between exterior and interior syndromes, cold and heat syndromes, deficiency and excess syndromes, Yin and Yang syndromes, and others.

For example, in a patient with pathogenic heat obstructing the lungs, initial symptoms may include high fever, flushed face, restlessness, and a rapid, forceful pulse. These manifestations reflect the vigorous response of the body's functional activities and are termed Yang syndrome, heat syndrome, and excess syndrome. However, as the disease progresses to a severe stage, due to the overwhelming accumulation of pathogenic heat and substantial depletion of the body's righteous Qi, the patient may suddenly exhibit signs of Yin and cold crisis, such as pale complexion, cold limbs, mental fatigue, and a faint, almost imperceptible pulse, despite the ongoing high fever, flushed face, restlessness, and rapid, forceful pulse. These signs indicate a failure in the body's adaptive capabilities and are termed Yin syndrome, cold syndrome, and deficiency syndrome.

Between blood and Qi, blood is considered Yin, and Qi is considered Yang. Within the category of Qi, Ying Qi (nutritive Qi) inside the body is Yin, and Wei Qi (defensive Qi) outside the body is Yang.

Excessive Yang manifests as a pathological increase of Yang pathogenic factors leading to a heat-related pathology. When a pathogenic factor, such as summer heat, invades the human body, it can cause an excessive accumulation of Yang Qi, resulting in symptoms like high fever, sweating, thirst, flushed face, and a rapid pulse. These manifestations are characterized by heat, hence the saying, "Excessive Yang leads to heat."

Excessive Yin, on the other hand, represents a pathological increase of Yin pathogenic factors leading to a cold-related pathology. When a pathogenic factor, such as exposure to cold or consumption of cold food, affects the body, it can cause an excessive accumulation of Yin Qi, resulting in symptoms like abdominal pain, diarrhea, cold limbs, pale tongue with a white coating, and a deep pulse. These manifestations are characterized by cold, hence the saying, "Excessive Yin leads to cold."

If the body's Yang Qi is weakened, symptoms may include a pale complexion, aversion to cold with cold limbs, fatigue leading to curling up, spontaneous sweating, and a faint pulse. The nature of these manifestations is also cold, hence the term "Deficient Yang leads to cold."

On the other hand, in cases of prolonged illness causing Yin depletion or inherent Yin deficiency, symptoms may include tidal fever, night sweats, restlessness with a feeling of heat in the chest, dry mouth and tongue, and a rapid, thin pulse. The nature of these manifestations is also heat, hence the term "Deficient Yin leads to heat."

The relationship between Qi and the Five Elements involves the differentiation of original Qi into the Five Elements, and the convergence of the Five Elements back into a unified Qi. The five material elements—metal, wood, water, fire, and earth—are formed through the movement and transformation of Qi.

According to the Five Elements theory, the internal organs of the human body are categorized under the Five Elements, and the characteristics of the Five Elements are used to explain the physiological functions of these organs. For example: Wood has a flexible and straight nature, smooth and unobstructed, and possesses the characteristics of growth and development. Therefore, the Liver favors smoothness and dislikes stagnation, demonstrating its function of promoting free flow. Fire has a warm and hot nature, and the Heart, attributed to fire, has the function of warming and providing warmth. Earth has a nurturing and grounding nature, and the Spleen, attributed to earth, is responsible for the digestion of grains, transportation of essence, and nourishing the organs, limbs, and bones, serving as the source of Qi and blood transformation. Metal has a clear and contracting nature, and the Lungs, attributed to metal, exhibit a clear and contracting quality, with the ability to disseminate and descend. Water has a moistening and downward nature, with characteristics of cold moisture, downward movement, and storage. The Kidneys, attributed to water, govern storage, hold essence, and regulate water functions.

Using the concept of the Five Elements generating each other, we can illustrate the connections between the internal organs. For example, Wood generates Fire, meaning the Liver's Wood supports the Heart's Fire. Since the Liver stores blood and the Heart governs the blood vessels, the normal function of blood storage in the Liver contributes to the normal functioning of the Heart in managing the blood vessels. Fire generates Earth, which implies that the Heart's Fire warms the Spleen's Earth. The Heart governs the blood vessels and mental activities, while the Spleen is responsible for transformation and production, as well as governing the blood and supporting the blood lineage. When the Heart's blood vessels function normally, the blood can nourish the Spleen, allowing it to carry out its functions of transformation, blood production, and blood regulation. Earth generates Metal, indicating that the Spleen's Earth assists the Lungs' Metal. The Spleen can tonify Qi, generate Qi and blood, transport essence to nourish the Lungs, and promote the Lungs' function of governing Qi, ensuring its normal operation. Metal generates Water, meaning the Lungs' Metal nourishes the Kidneys' Water. The Lungs govern purification, and the Kidneys store essence. The Lungs' clear descending function aids the Kidneys in storing essence, receiving Qi, and governing water. Water generates Wood, indicating that the Kidneys' Water nourishes the Liver's Wood. The Kidneys store essence, the Liver stores blood, and the Kidneys' essence can transform into Liver's blood, contributing to the normal function of the Liver.

In summary, Traditional Chinese Medicine, following the logical structure of Qi – Yin and Yang – Five Elements, elucidates the fundamental laws of life processes and establishes the theoretical framework of Chinese medicine based on the contradictory movement of Qi, Yin and Yang, and the Five Elements.

# Chapter 3

## The Human Organs In TCM Terms

The term "visceral manifestation" primarily refers to the signs of organ function activities within the human body. The theory of visceral manifestations studies the morphological structure, physiological activity patterns, and their interrelations of the organs and orifices. It posits that the human body centers around the five viscera—heart, liver, spleen, lung, and kidney—complemented by the six bowels—gallbladder, stomach, large intestine, small intestine, bladder, and triple burner (sanjiao), with qi, blood, essence, and body fluids as the material basis. This forms five functional activity systems that internally connect the five viscera and six bowels and externally to the body's orifices and structures.

The term "viscera and bowels" collectively refers to the five viscera, six bowels, and the "extraordinary organs" (brain, marrow, bones, vessels, gallbladder, and the female uterus).

From a functional perspective, the five viscera primarily govern the "storage of essence and qi," meaning they are responsible for the synthesis and storage of vital substances such as qi, blood, body fluids, and essence. They oversee complex life processes, ensuring the abundance of these substances.

The six bowels, on the other hand, serve the function of "transforming and transporting substances." They receive and digest grains and liquids, transforming and excreting waste materials. Their main role is in the digestion, absorption, transportation, and elimination of ingested food. They are characterized by being full but not capable of storage.

The extraordinary organs, characterized by various cavities, are closely related to the bowels. They serve the function of storing essence and qi, resembling both viscera and bowels. Though they seem like viscera and bowels, they are neither entirely viscera nor bowels. They are stored in the yin aspect and resemble the earth, thus remaining hidden without discharge.

The holistic perspective centered around the five viscera is a fundamental characteristic of the theory of visceral manifestations. The research focus of this theory is the living and vital human being. The human body is an extremely complex organic whole with the five viscera at its core. The various components of the human body are inseparable in terms of morphological structure, harmoniously coordinated in physiological functions, interlinked in material metabolism, and mutually influential in pathology.

Here, I will only discuss the primary functions of the five viscera and six bowels.

## The Five Viscera

### Heart

The heart, classified as Fire in the Five Elements, is the supreme yang organ among yang organs. It governs the blood vessels, houses the spirit and consciousness, and acts as the primary master and ruler of life among the five viscera and six bowels.

In Traditional Chinese Medicine, the pulsation of the pulse is examined through touch to understand the overall state of qi and blood in the body, serving as one of the diagnostic foundations known as "pulse diagnosis." Under normal physiological conditions, when the heart functions properly, and qi and blood circulate smoothly, the pulse rhythm is even, gentle, and strong.

With a normal functioning heart, the heartbeat is regular, the pulse is even, and the rhythm is harmonious, leading to a rosy and lustrous complexion. If there is a pathological change in the heart, it will be reflected through aspects such as heartbeats, pulse, and complexion. For instance, insufficient heart qi, deficient blood, or obstructed pulse channels may result in poor blood circulation, a pale complexion, and a weak pulse. In severe cases, blood stasis and obstruction of blood vessels may lead to a dusky complexion, bluish lips and tongue, chest oppression, stabbing pain in the precordial region, and irregular, hesitant, rapid, or rough pulses.

The heart governs the spirit and consciousness. While each of the five viscera has its own domain, the primary physiological function of governing the spirit and consciousness belongs to the heart.

The heart governs the blood, supplying it to the brain. Therefore, the heart and brain are closely connected, often mentioned together, and work together in harmony.

When the physiological function of the heart in governing the spirit and consciousness is normal, the individual experiences mental alertness, clear consciousness, sharp thinking, and a sensitive and normal response to external stimuli. If there is an abnormality in the physiological function of the heart in governing the spirit and consciousness, it can lead to various mental disturbances such as insomnia, vivid dreams, restlessness, and even delirium. Other manifestations may include delayed reactions, mental lethargy, and in severe cases, unconsciousness and loss of awareness. Moreover, these abnormalities can impact the functions of other organs and may even pose a threat to the entire life.

**Lungs**

The lungs, residing above the diaphragm along with the heart, are connected to the trachea, open to the nose, and directly communicate with the ambient atmosphere. They form the pulmonary system along with the large intestine, skin, hair, and nose. In the context of the Five Elements, the lungs belong to the metal element and are the yin organ within yang. They govern qi, oversee respiration, assist the heart in circulating blood, and regulate the water passages. Among the five viscera and six bowels, the lungs are positioned at the highest level, serving as the chief among the five viscera.

The lungs participate in the generation of the body's qi, particularly the ancestral qi. Through respiratory movements, the lungs inhale the clear qi from the natural environment. Simultaneously, through the digestive and absorptive functions of the gastrointestinal tract, ingested food is transformed into vital essence. The spleen then raises the clear aspect, transporting it upward to the lungs. The clear qi from the natural environment and the vital essence from food combine within the lungs, accumulating in the upper sea of qi within the chest, known as ancestral qi. Ancestral qi rises to the throat, promoting respiratory movements, and travels through the heart's meridians to circulate blood and qi throughout the body, warming and nourishing the organs and tissues to maintain their normal functions.

The respiratory movements of the lungs are a specific manifestation of the ascending and descending inhalation-exhalation motions of qi. The rhythmic inhalation and exhalation of the lungs play a crucial role in regulating the overall ascending and descending movements of qi in the body.

The lungs govern the circulation of water, indicating their role in facilitating and regulating the distribution, movement, and excretion of bodily fluids. The metabolism of bodily fluids is a collaborative effort among the lungs, spleen, kidneys, as well as the small intestine, large intestine, bladder, and other organs.

Only when the lung qi functions normally in both spreading and descending can it allow the smooth flow of qi, ensuring unobstructed airways, even breathing, and maintaining the exchange of gases inside and outside the body. This ensures that various organs and tissues receive nourishment from qi, blood, and body fluids, while preventing the retention of dampness, phlegm, and impurities. This balanced function of lung qi prevents excessive dissipation, maintaining a consistently clear and normal state.

When lung qi fails in its dispersing function, symptoms such as difficulty breathing, chest tightness, coughing, as well as nasal congestion, sneezing, and lack of perspiration may occur.

The physiological function of the lungs is most susceptible to the influence of external environmental factors. Particularly, pathogenic factors like wind and cold tend to invade the lungs first, leading to disorders such as a loss of lung-wei function and impediment of lung orifices. Since the lungs are closely related to the skin and hair, initial manifestations of such disorders often include symptoms like fever, chills, and coughing; nasal congestion is also common when lung-wei function is disrupted.

During autumn, the dry pathogenic influence easily invades the human body and depletes the lung's yin and moisture, resulting in symptoms such as dry cough, dry skin, and dryness of the mouth and nose. Additionally, conditions like wind-cold binding the surface can invade the lung-wei, causing symptoms of aversion to cold, fever, severe headache, and a floating pulse, indicating an externally contracted condition.

### Spleen

The spleen, along with the stomach, flesh, lips, and mouth, constitutes the spleen system. It is primarily responsible for transportation and transformation, controlling blood, distributing the essence of food and drink, and serving as the source of qi and blood generation. The spleen moistens and nourishes all organs and parts of the body, hence it is known as the foundation of postnatal existence.

The spleen's role in transportation and transformation refers to its ability to process food and drink into their essence and to distribute this essential substance throughout the body's organs and tissues.

After food is digested and absorbed, its essence is transported and spread by the spleen upwards to the lungs, from where it is sent into the heart meridian to be transformed into qi and blood. This is then circulated throughout the body via the meridians, nourishing the organs, limbs, skin, muscles, and other tissues and organs.

Only when the spleen's qi is robust and functioning properly can the body's digestive and absorptive functions be sound. This ensures an ample supply of nutrients for the generation of qi, blood, and body fluids, providing comprehensive nourishment to all organs and tissues throughout the body to maintain normal physiological activities. Conversely, if the spleen's function is compromised, the digestive and absorptive capabilities of the body become irregular, leading to pathological changes such as abdominal bloating, loose stools, loss of appetite, fatigue, emaciation, and insufficient qi and blood.

When the spleen's ability to transform and transport dampness is healthy, it not only ensures adequate moisture for all tissues in the body but also prevents excessive retention of dampness. On the contrary, if the spleen's function in transforming and transporting dampness is impaired, it will inevitably result in stagnation of fluids within the body, giving rise to pathological products like dampness and phlegm, and in severe cases, leading to the formation of edema.

The spleen's transformation of food essence includes the generation of blood through the process of qi transformation. When the spleen's qi is robust and functioning well, there is an ample supply of transformative energy, leading to abundant qi and blood. If the spleen's function is compromised, resulting in a deficiency of the materials needed for blood generation, blood deficiency occurs, leading to symptoms such as dizziness, blurred vision, and signs of blood deficiency such as paleness in the face, lips, tongue, and nails.

The spleen governs blood, and when the spleen is deficient, it cannot properly control blood. Due to the weakened spleen function and depleted yang qi, it fails to control the blood flow, leading to a condition known as "spleen failing to govern blood." Clinically, this manifests as subcutaneous bleeding, gastrointestinal bleeding, hematuria, and abnormal uterine bleeding, with lower part bleeding being particularly common.

The spleen's role in managing dampness is adversely affected when the spleen is overwhelmed by dampness. If the spleen is hindered by dampness and its function is impaired, it can result in symptoms such as fullness and distention in the chest and abdomen, reduced appetite, fatigue, loose and thin stools, a sweet taste in the mouth with excessive salivation, and a greasy tongue coating. These symptoms reflect the relationship between the spleen and dampness.

**Liver**

The liver, together with the gallbladder, eyes, tendons, and nails, forms the liver system. It is primarily responsible for dispersion and excretion, storing blood, preferring expression and detesting suppression, and utilizing yin to wield yang.

The liver's role in dispersion refers to its ability to ensure the smooth flow of the body's qi, maintaining unobstructed and smooth circulation throughout, thereby preventing stagnation and congestion.

The liver's dispersion function plays a crucial role in regulating and maintaining the balance and coordination of the qi movement across all organs and tissues of the body, including the ascending, descending, entering, and exiting of qi.

Through its dispersion function, the liver plays a role in regulating emotional activities and mood. The liver's role in planning and deliberation aids the heart in regulating cognitive and emotional activities. Under normal physiological conditions, if the liver's dispersion function is normal and liver qi ascends properly without being overly excited or suppressed, one can better coordinate their emotional activities, resulting in a pleasant mood, emotional well-being, clear reasoning, and sharp thinking, with balanced qi and blood. However, if the liver fails to disperse properly, it can lead to abnormalities in emotional activities. Inadequate dispersion manifests as depression, melancholy, and excessive worry. Excessive dispersion results in irritability, headaches, and red eyes.

The liver's promotion of the digestive and absorptive functions of the spleen and stomach is achieved through coordinating the ascending and descending movements of their qi and through the secretion and excretion of bile.

If the liver fails in its dispersion function and negatively impacts the spleen and stomach, it leads to irregularities in their ascending and descending movements. Clinically, aside from symptoms of liver qi stagnation, one may experience disharmony between the liver and stomach, resulting in symptoms such as warmth and fullness in the epigastrium due to the failure of stomach qi to descend, nausea, and reduced appetite. Additionally, symptoms of liver-spleen disharmony, such as abdominal distension and loose stools due to the failure of spleen qi to ascend, may also manifest.

When the liver's dispersion function is normal, bile is secreted and excreted properly, aiding in the digestive and absorptive functions of the spleen and stomach. However, if liver qi stagnation affects bile secretion and excretion, it can lead to digestive absorption disorders, resulting in symptoms such as rib pain, bitter taste in the mouth, indigestion, and even jaundice.

The liver's dispersion function directly influences the smooth flow of qi. Only when the qi flows smoothly can the heart effectively govern blood vessels, the lungs assist in the circulation of blood, and the spleen control and manage blood circulation. This ensures the normal circulation of qi and blood.

The liver regulates the body's water metabolism through its function of dispersing, benefiting, and harmonizing the qi of the three burners and organs. This forms the theoretical basis of "regulating water by promoting qi."

If the liver fails in its dispersion function, leading to a disharmony of the Chong and Ren channels, it can result in menstrual disorders, abnormal vaginal discharge, issues related to pregnancy and childbirth, as well as sexual dysfunction and infertility.

When the liver's dispersion function is in harmony with the kidney's storing function, the opening and closing of the essence chamber are appropriately regulated, and the excretion of semen is controlled. This ensures the normal sexual and reproductive functions in men. If the liver's dispersion function is impaired, it can lead to imbalances in opening and closing and excretion. Inadequate dispersion may manifest as decreased libido, impotence, low semen volume, and infertility, while excessive dispersion can lead to heightened sexual desire, strong erections, and nocturnal emissions.

The liver stores a certain amount of blood, serving to nourish itself, regulate the balance of liver yin and yang, maintain the harmony of qi and blood, and prevent excessive bleeding.

When individuals are in a state of quiet rest and emotional stability, as the activity levels of various body parts decrease, the demand for peripheral blood also decreases. Consequently, a portion of the blood returns to be stored in the liver. This is known as "when people move, blood circulates through the meridians; when people are still, blood returns to the liver." Due to its function of storing and regulating blood volume, the liver is referred to as the "Sea of Blood."

Physiologically, the liver stores blood, and the nourishment from the blood helps maintain a balanced liver yang, ensuring the normal function of the liver's dispersion. In pathological conditions, insufficient blood storage in the liver or bleeding from the liver leads to a deficiency of liver blood. When there is insufficient liver blood, the liver is not adequately nourished, and the dispersion function is impaired, resulting in symptoms such as restless sleep, vivid dreams, and irregular menstruation in women.

When liver blood is deficient, the blood distributed throughout the body cannot meet the physiological needs, leading to pathological changes associated with blood deficiency. For instance, if the eyes lack blood nourishment, it may result in dryness, blurred vision, or even night blindness. If the tendons lack nourishment, symptoms such as stiffness, numbness, difficulty in bending or stretching limbs, reduced menstrual flow in women, and even amenorrhea may occur. The absence of blood storage in the liver can lead to pathological changes with a tendency for bleeding, such as vomiting blood, nosebleeds, excessive menstruation, and metrorrhagia.

Liver blood deficiency may manifest as symptoms such as muscle spasms, arching of the fingers and toes, seizures, withering of the nails, dizziness, headaches, rib-side pain, lower abdominal pain, and hernia pain.

When liver qi ascends excessively, symptoms such as irritability, anger, dizziness, and headaches may arise.

In terms of pathological changes in the liver, there is a tendency towards hyperactivity of yang and susceptibility to internal wind disturbances. Liver diseases often manifest as liver yang hyperactivity and internal liver wind movement, resulting in symptoms such as dizziness, numbness in the limbs, convulsions, tremors, and arching of the fingers and toes.

**Kidneys**

The kidneys, along with the bladder, bone marrow, brain, hair, and ears, constitute the kidney system. They govern the storage of essence, control bodily fluids, and master the reception of qi. The kidneys are regarded as the foundation of Yin and Yang in the body's organs, representing the source of life and are therefore referred to as the foundation of congenital essence.

Congenital essence can only fully exert its physiological effects when supplemented and nourished by acquired essence. Similarly, acquired essence can maintain its vitality only with the support of congenital essence.

The Huangdi Neijing (Yellow Emperor's Inner Canon) makes it clear that after birth, through the mutual nourishment of congenital and acquired essences, the essence and energy of the kidneys gradually become abundant. As a person develops from childhood to adolescence, the essence of the kidneys continuously flourishes. In the youth period, with the constant enrichment of kidney essence, a substance promoting the maturation of reproductive functions called Tian Gui (Heavenly Water) is produced. As a result, males can generate semen, and females experience regular menstrual cycles, marking the gradual maturation of reproductive capabilities.

The ebb and flow of the organs and vital energy in the human body follow a pattern of prosperity, decline, and depletion with the increase in age.

If kidney essence is deficient, it can affect the growth and development of the body, leading to developmental issues such as delayed growth and weakened muscles and bones. In adulthood, premature aging may manifest with symptoms like shaky teeth and hair loss.

The kidneys store essence, and this essence can give rise to marrow, which, in turn, can transform into blood. Kidney essence plays a role in resisting external pathogens and protecting the body from diseases.

The kidneys govern bodily fluids. In a broad sense, this refers to the kidneys as the "water organ," indicating their role in storing essence and regulating bodily fluids. In a narrow sense, it signifies the kidneys' function in overseeing and regulating the metabolism of bodily fluids in the human body.

The steaming and transformation of the kidneys allow other organs like the lungs, spleen, and bladder to play their respective physiological roles in the metabolism of bodily fluids. The water and fluids utilized by organ tissues (the turbid within the clear) descend from the Triple Burner to return to the kidneys. Through the kidney's transformative function, these fluids are separated into clear and turbid components. The clear part ascends through the Triple Burner and returns to the lungs, where it disperses throughout the body. The turbid part transforms into urine, descends to the bladder, and is excreted through the urethra. This cycle repeats to maintain the balance of the body's fluid metabolism. The kidney's transformative function is a central aspect in regulating the balance of fluid metabolism.

When the kidney's water-regulating function is disrupted, and transformative processes are compromised, it can lead to disorders in fluid metabolism. Abnormal transformative processes, inadequate closing of the gates, or excessive opening can result in urinary issues, leading to pathologies such as reduced urine output, edema, increased urine output, and frequent urination.

The kidneys govern the inhalation of qi, playing a crucial role in the body's respiratory movements. Only when kidney qi is abundant and inhalation is normal can the lungs ensure smooth and even breathing with unobstructed airways. If the kidney's function of inhaling qi diminishes, and it cannot properly absorb the inhaled air, leading to the inability to incorporate the absorbed qi into the kidneys, pathological changes such as rapid exhalation, difficulty inhaling, and pronounced breathlessness may occur.

The relationship between kidney yin and yang forms the foundation of the yin and yang in the organs. Deficiency of kidney yin manifests as symptoms like internal heat, dizziness, tinnitus, soreness and weakness in the lower back and knees, nocturnal emissions in men, and dream-disturbed sleep in women. Deficiency of kidney yang presents with fatigue, cold and painful lower back and knees, cold limbs, urinary difficulties or incontinence, as well as impotence in men, infertility in women due to uterine cold, and symptoms of edema.

The essence of the kidneys should not be depleted, and the kidney's fire should not be excessively suppressed. It is likened to the roots of a tree and the source of water: just as the roots of a tree should not be severed, and the water source should not be exhausted, nurturing the roots leads to flourishing branches and leaves, and purifying the water source results in clarity. Therefore, the physiological characteristic of the kidneys is to store and not to excessively deplete, as reflected in the functions of storing essence, inhaling qi, controlling water, and securing pregnancy.

## The Six Fu Organs

The Six Fu (or Fu organs) , also called the Six Bowels, refer to the gallbladder, stomach, small intestine, large intestine, bladder, and triple heater (sanjiao). When food and drink enter the body, they pass through the esophagus into the stomach. After undergoing fermentation in the stomach, the partially digested contents move to the small intestine. In the small intestine, the clear (nutrients and fluids) are absorbed by the spleen, transferred to the lungs, and distributed throughout the body to support the needs of the organs, meridians, and overall life activities. The impurities (residue) continue to the large intestine, where they are further processed and expelled as feces. Waste liquids are transformed into urine by the qi transformation of the kidneys, filtering into the bladder before being expelled from the body.

The physiological characteristics of the Six Bowel Organs involve storage and transformation of water and grains. They handle the intake of food and drink; the stomach is responsible for fermentation, the small intestine for separation of clear and turbid substances, the spleen for absorption, the large intestine for elimination of feces, and the bladder for urine storage and elimination. Each organ must timely empty its contents to maintain the smooth functioning and coordination of the Six Bowels.

### Gallbladder

Gallbladder, in conjunction with the liver, is considered as a paired organ with an interior-exterior relationship. The liver belongs to the yin wood category as a zang (solid) organ, while the gallbladder belongs to the yang wood category as a fu (hollow) organ. The gallbladder stores and excretes bile, governs decision-making, and regulates the qi of the zang-fu organs. The gallbladder is considered a pure organ, favoring tranquility and disliking agitation.

Bile is produced and secreted by the liver, then stored and concentrated in the gallbladder. Through the gallbladder's excretory function, bile enters the small intestine to aid in the digestion and absorption of food, facilitating the smooth passage of waste. If there is insufficient bile, the distinction between the pure and impure components becomes unclear, resulting in pale and clean feces without the typical yellow color.

If the functions of the liver and gallbladder are impaired, leading to obstruction of bile secretion and excretion, it can affect the digestive functions of the spleen and stomach, resulting in symptoms of poor digestion such as loss of appetite, abdominal distension, and diarrhea. If dampness and heat accumulate in the liver and gallbladder, causing the liver to lose its dispersing and excreting functions and the overflow of bile, it may lead to jaundice, characterized by yellowing of the eyes, skin, and urine. When bile descends smoothly, there is a normal flow, but if bile circulation is hindered, it can lead to bitter taste in the mouth, vomiting of bitter and greenish fluids, and other symptoms.

Psychological and mental activities are related to the decision-making function of the gallbladder, as the gallbladder assists the liver in dispersing and regulating emotions. When the liver and gallbladder work in harmony, emotions are stable. Individuals with a robust gallbladder can withstand intense mental stimuli with relatively little impact, and they recover quickly. Therefore, it is said that a strong gallbladder is resistant to external pathogenic factors. People with a weak gallbladder, when exposed to adverse psychological stimuli, are more prone to developing illnesses, manifesting as timidity, easy startle, fearfulness, insomnia, and vivid dreams, among other mental and emotional disturbances.

**Stomach**

The stomach is an organ in the abdominal cavity that accommodates food. It has a curved shape, connected to the esophagus above and leading to the small intestine below. Its main function is to receive and ripen cereals and water, serving as a repository for refined grains and a sea of qi and blood. The stomach functions to descend and pass through, cooperating with the spleen, and the spleen-stomach are often collectively referred to as the foundation of postnatal essence. While both the stomach and spleen reside in the central earth, the stomach, being dry earth, is yang, while the spleen, being damp earth, is yin.

The receiving function of the stomach is the basis for its ripening function and the foundation of the entire digestive process. If the stomach is affected by pathology, it can impact its receiving function, leading to symptoms such as poor appetite, aversion to food, and distension in the epigastric region.

After food is preliminarily digested, the refined substances are transformed and nourish the entire body through the spleen's processing. Undigested food particles descend to the small intestine, undergoing continuous renewal, forming the digestive process of the stomach. If the stomach's ripening function is compromised, symptoms of stomach pain in the epigastric region and regurgitation of foul-smelling food due to food stagnation may occur.

The stomach's functions of receiving and ripening cereals and water must be coordinated with the spleen's transforming function to be successfully carried out. The spleen should ascend for health, while the stomach should descend for harmony. When the spleen ascends and the stomach descends, they coordinate with each other, working together to complete the digestion and absorption of food.

The strength or weakness of stomach qi is closely related to the vital activities and survival of the human body. In the course of human life activities, it holds significant importance.

Stomach qi can manifest in aspects such as appetite, tongue coating, pulse, and facial complexion. Generally, when the appetite is normal, the tongue coating is normal, the facial complexion is vibrant, and the pulse is steady and moderate (neither too fast nor too slow), it is considered to have stomach qi. In clinical practice, the presence or absence of stomach qi is often used as an important basis for judging the prognosis, where the presence of stomach qi signifies life, and the absence of stomach qi signifies death. Protecting stomach qi essentially involves safeguarding the functions of the spleen and stomach.

The stomach's ability to receive and ripen relies not only on the warming function of stomach yang but also on the moistening effect of gastric fluids. Only when there is sufficient gastric fluid can the stomach digest cereals and maintain its descending and downward-moving nature. As the stomach is a yang earth organ that prefers moisture over dryness, its ailments tend to develop into dry-heat damage, particularly harming stomach yin. Therefore, in the treatment of stomach disorders, attention should be paid to protecting stomach yin. Even if the use of bitter and cold purgatives is necessary, it should be done cautiously and discontinued promptly, aiming to eliminate excessive heat and dryness without indiscriminately employing bitter and cold remedies to avoid further damage to yin caused by dryness.

### Small Intestine

The small intestine is located in the abdominal cavity, connecting to the pylorus above and communicating with the stomach. It extends downward to the large intestine, including the ileum, jejunum, and duodenum. The small intestine is responsible for digesting and separating clear from turbid substances. It is associated with the heart, both belonging to the fire element and having a yang nature.

After initial digestion in the stomach, dietary substances must stay in the small intestine for a certain period. The small intestine further digests and absorbs these substances, transforming cereals and water into usable nutrients. The essence is extracted, while the residues pass into the large intestine.

In pathological conditions, if the small intestine's function of containing and transforming is disrupted, the flow of qi becomes obstructed, leading to stagnation and pain, manifested as abdominal pain. Dysfunction in the transformation process can result in digestive and absorptive disorders, leading to symptoms such as abdominal distension, diarrhea, and loose stools.

The small intestine transports the residual waste and impurities of ingested food through the ileocecal valve into the large intestine, forming feces that are expelled from the body through the anus. It also filters the remaining water, which undergoes vaporization in the kidneys before entering the bladder as urine, ultimately being expelled from the body through the urethra.

When the small intestine's functions are disrupted, the distinction between clear and turbid substances becomes unclear, leading to a mixture of fluids and solid waste, resulting in symptoms such as loose stools and diarrhea. Dysfunction in the separation of clear and turbid substances not only affects bowel movements but also impacts urination, leading to decreased urine output.

When there is poor digestion and absorption in the small intestine, it falls within the scope of spleen deficiency, often requiring treatment based on the principles of the spleen and stomach. The ascending of clear and descending of turbid functions in the small intestine are concrete manifestations of the spleen's ascending clear and the stomach's descending turbid functions. When these functions are disrupted, leading to a lack of separation between clear and turbid substances, symptoms such as vomiting, abdominal distension, and diarrhea may occur.

**Large Intestine**

The large intestine is located in the abdominal cavity, with its upper opening connected to the small intestine at the ileocecal valve and its lower end closely linked to the anus. It includes the colon and rectum and is primarily responsible for transforming waste and absorbing fluid. In the context of the body's organ relationships, it is associated with the lungs, belonging to the metal element and having a yang nature.

The main function of the large intestine is to transport waste and eliminate feces. Its transporting function is closely related to the descending function of the stomach, the transforming function of the spleen, the descending and purging function of the lungs, and the sealing and storing function of the kidneys.

When the large intestine is affected, and its transporting function is disrupted, it is mainly manifested by changes in the quantity and quality of stools and alterations in bowel movement frequency. Abnormalities in large intestine transportation can lead to conditions such as constipation or diarrhea. If damp-heat accumulates in the large intestine, causing stagnation of colon qi, symptoms like abdominal pain, urgency followed by heaviness, and bloody or purulent diarrhea may occur.

After receiving food residues and remaining water from the small intestine, the large intestine reabsorbs some of the water, allowing the formation of feces, which are then expelled from the body.

A deficient and cold large intestine is unable to efficiently absorb water, resulting in the passage of mixed substances, leading to symptoms such as bowel sounds, abdominal pain, and diarrhea. Conversely, a large intestine with excess heat evaporates water, causing dryness in the intestinal fluid and loss of lubrication, leading to symptoms of constipation and obstruction.

**Bladder**

The bladder is primarily responsible for storing and excreting urine and is internally-externally related to the kidneys. In the Five Elements, it belongs to water and its nature is yang.

In the process of body fluid metabolism, fluids are distributed throughout the body by the lungs, spleen, and kidneys, playing a role in moisturizing the body.

Urine is stored in the bladder and, when it reaches a certain volume, the vaporizing action of the kidneys allows the bladder to open and close appropriately, so that urine can be timely expelled from the body through the urinary orifice.

Urine and body fluids often affect each other; if there is a lack of body fluids, then there will be scanty urination; conversely, excessive urination can also lead to the loss of body fluids.

Bladder disorders are often related to the kidneys, and clinical treatment of abnormal urination often starts with the kidneys. The vaporization function of the bladder, in reality, belongs to the vaporizing action of the kidneys. If the kidney's function of consolidation and vaporization is abnormal, then the vaporizing function of the bladder is disrupted, losing its ability to properly open and close, which can lead to difficulties in urination or urinary retention, as well as symptoms like frequent urination, urgent urination, incontinence, and inability to hold urine.

**The Three Burners**

The collective term for the Upper Burner (Shangjiao), Middle Burner (Zhongjiao), and Lower Burner (Xiaojiao) is one of the six Fu organs and is the largest among the Zang-Fu organs. It is also referred to as the External Fu or the Solitary Organ. Its main functions include promoting the ascending and descending movements of various Qi and facilitating the circulation of fluids. In the Five Elements, it is associated with fire, and its Yin-Yang nature is yang.

The Upper Burner includes the heart and lungs; the Middle Burner includes the spleen and stomach; and the Lower Burner includes the liver, kidneys, small intestine, bladder, and the uterus in women. Although the liver is anatomically associated with the Middle Burner, it is grouped with the kidneys in the Lower Burner due to their close relationship. The functions of the Triple Burner essentially represent the overall functions of all the Zang-Fu organs.

The primordial Qi flows through the Triple Burner and distributes to the Zang-Fu organs, nourishing the entire body and stimulating the functional activities of various organ tissues. Therefore, the Triple Burner is considered the pathway for the circulation of primordial Qi.

The lungs in the Upper Burner serve as the source of water, disseminating and descending to regulate the water passages. The spleen and stomach in the Middle Burner transform and distribute fluids to the lungs. The kidneys and bladder in the Lower Burner steam and vaporize, allowing fluids to ascend to the spleen and lungs, participating in internal metabolism, and ultimately forming urine that is expelled from the body. The Triple Burner functions as the pathway for the generation, distribution, ascending, descending, and excretion of fluids.

The Triple Burner has the function of transforming water and grains, assisting in digestion and absorption, and plays a role in circulating fluids, distributing refined substances, and eliminating waste.

### The Six Unique Organs

The brain, marrow, bones, vessels, gallbladder, and the uterus in women are collectively referred to as the "Qiheng Zhi Fu" (strange and unique organs).

The brain, when combined with the skull, is called the head. The head occupies the highest point of the human body and is the dwelling place of the spirit. The Qi and blood of the twelve meridians and three hundred and sixty-five collaterals all converge in the head. Therefore, the head is referred to as the gathering place of all yang energies, the location of the clear orifices, where the clear and yang Qi of the human body ascend.

The brain is considered the residence of the Yuan Shen (◇◇), the primary spirit. The Yuan Shen is the pivotal force of life, and it is said,

"Pierce a person's brain, and the true Qi will dissipate, leading to instant death."

If the brain's function of governing mental consciousness is normal, one's spirit is full, consciousness is clear, thinking is sharp, memory is strong, language is clear, and emotions are normal.

The eyes, ears, mouth, nose, and tongue, as the external orifices of the five Zang organs, are all located in the head and face and are connected to the brain. Human functions such as vision, hearing, speech, and movement are all closely related to the brain.

When the brain is nourished and filled, the body feels light, energetic, and powerful. Otherwise, if there is deficiency, symptoms such as sore shins and impaired functionality may occur. Regardless of deficiency or excess, it can manifest as hearing loss, blurred vision, impaired sense of smell, and abnormal sensations.

The kidneys store essence, and essence generates marrow, which accumulates in the brain. Therefore, the physiological relationship between the brain and the kidneys is particularly close. When the kidney essence is abundant and the marrow is nourished, the brain develops soundly, resulting in abundant energy, keen hearing and vision, agile thinking, and dexterous movements. If the kidney essence is deficient, the marrow lacks nourishment, and the brain marrow is insufficient, symptoms such as dizziness, forgetfulness, and tinnitus may occur. In severe cases, there may be memory decline and sluggish thinking.

If the lungs function normally, Qi is abundant, and the marrow receives ample nourishment. Therefore, there is a close relationship between the brain and the lungs. Consequently, in clinical practice, brain disorders can be treated from the perspective of the lungs.

**Marrow**

Marrow is a paste-like substance in the bone cavity, collectively referring to the brain marrow, spinal marrow, and bone marrow. Marrow is generated from the congenital essence and nourished by the acquired essence, with the functions of nourishing the brain, enriching the bones, and transforming into blood.

When the brain receives nourishment from the marrow and is filled with brain marrow, resulting in abundant mental energy, the functions of the primordial spirit are vigorous, leading to keen hearing, clear vision, and a strong, healthy body.

Marrow is stored within bones, and bones rely on marrow for nourishment. When bones are nourished by bone marrow, they grow and develop normally, maintaining their firmness and strength. If kidney essence is deficient, leading to a lack of nourishment for the bone marrow, this can result in fragile, weak bones or poor development.

Essence and blood can generate each other; essence generates marrow, and marrow can also transform into blood. In cases of blood deficiency, treatment often involves methods to nourish the kidney and replenish essence.

### The Uterus

The uterus, also known as the womb or "nü zibao" (◇◇◇), is situated in the central lower abdomen and serves as the internal reproductive organ in females. It plays a crucial role in overseeing menstruation and nurturing a developing fetus.

Menstruation is a physiological phenomenon characterized by periodic uterine bleeding after the maturation of female reproductive cells. In healthy females, reproductive organ development is completed around the age of 14, and the uterus undergoes cyclic changes, resulting in approximately monthly episodes of uterine bleeding. Menstruation typically begins around the age of 14 and continues until around 49 years of age. The blood in the uterus is refreshed monthly, representing a renewal process.

The uterus is the organ responsible for pregnancy and childbirth in females. After reaching reproductive maturity, females have the ability to conceive when menstruation occurs timely.

In the context of the Five Zang organs, the relationship between the uterus and the liver, spleen, and kidneys is particularly significant. The liver is considered the sea of blood, storing and governing blood, serving as the foundation for women's menstrual cycles. The connection between the uterus and the spleen is mainly manifested in two aspects: the transformation and generation of menstrual blood and the consolidation and vaporization of menstrual blood. When the spleen's Qi is robust, the sources for transformation are sufficient, and governance is in order, resulting in normal retention and discharge of menstrual blood. As women enter old age, the decline in kidney essence and the depletion of the natural endowment lead to the cessation of menstruation, and reproductive capacity is gradually lost.

## The Five Tissue Structures, The Five Senses and The Nine Orifices

The five types of tissues—blood vessels, tendons, muscles, skin, and bones—are collectively referred to as the "Five Tissue Structures." Each of the five Zang organs governs a specific type of tissue: the heart governs blood vessels, the lungs govern the skin, the liver governs tendons, the spleen governs muscles, and the kidneys govern bones. The five sensory organs—the tongue, nose, mouth, eyes, and ears—are collectively referred to as the "Five Senses" or "Wu Guan."

There are seven orifices, collectively known as the "Seven Orifices" or "Qi Chuang," which include the eyes (two), ears (two), nostrils (two), and mouth. These orifices are located in the head and face. Additionally, there are two Yin orifices, referring to the front and back orifices.

### Blood Vessels

The blood vessels serve as the pathway for the circulation of Qi and blood. The pulse, as a relatively closed system of channels, permeates the entire body, reaching every corner, forming a dense network that encompasses the external muscles, skin, and hair, as well as the internal organs and cavities, creating an intricate network throughout the entire body.

The heart governs blood, the lungs govern Qi, and the pulse transports blood and Qi. Only when these three work together can the circulation of Qi and blood be completed.

After the digestion and absorption of food by the Middle Burner (spleen and stomach), water and grain essences are produced, which are then transported throughout the body via the blood vessels, providing ample nutrition for the physiological activities of various organs and viscera.

If the quantity of Qi and blood in the vessels is reduced, resulting in nutritional deficiency, it can lead to overall Qi and blood insufficiency. Abnormalities in the speed of Qi and blood circulation in the vessels, whether slow circulation leading to blood stasis or accelerated circulation causing reckless bleeding, can occur.

The abundance or deficiency of Qi and blood in the human body, as well as the strength or weakness of organ functions, can all be reflected through the pulse. Therefore, diagnosing diseases can be achieved by analyzing the pulse to infer pathological changes in the body.

### Skin

The skin serves as the body's outermost layer and plays multiple roles, including defending the body, resisting external pathogens, regulating fluid metabolism, controlling body temperature, and facilitating functions such as respiration and sensation.

The skin acts as a barrier to defend against external pathogens. The defensive Qi flows through the skin and hair, aiding the skin in protecting the body and functioning as a barrier against external pathogens. If the defensive Qi is weak, the skin becomes lax, and the pores open, making it easier for external pathogens to invade and cause illness.

Normal sweating serves to harmonize nutrient and defensive Qi, moisturizing the skin. By excreting sweat, the skin regulates body temperature to maintain a relatively constant level.

The lungs govern Qi, and lung Qi spreads to nourish the skin and hair by distributing defensive Qi, blood, and body fluids throughout the body.

If lung Qi is deficient, leading to weakened functions of spreading defensive Qi and transporting nutrients to the skin and hair, the ability to resist external pathogens is diminished, making individuals more susceptible to colds or displaying signs of withered and dry skin and hair.

In cases of lung Qi deficiency, where the protective layer of the skin is not solid, spontaneous sweating and weak breathing may occur. Additionally, if external pathogens attack the skin, pores may close, resulting in a lack of sweating and symptoms such as shortness of breath.

**Muscles**

All forms of movement in the human body require the coordinated effort of muscles, fascia, and joints, but it is primarily the contraction and relaxation activities of muscles that facilitate these movements.

Muscles not only serve to protect internal organs and cushion against external forces but also resist the invasion of external pathogens.

The nutrition of muscles comes from the water and grain essences absorbed and transported by the spleen. The strength and condition of the body's muscles are related to the spleen's digestive and transformative functions.

If the spleen's Qi is weak and there is nutritional deficiency, it will lead to thin and weak muscles, and even atrophy. The limbs of the human body rely on the spleen's Qi to transport nutrients to maintain their normal functional activities. When the spleen's Qi is robust and the nutrition is sufficient, the limbs are agile and strong. Conversely, if the spleen's Qi is deficient and there is inadequate nutrition, the limbs may feel tired, weak, or even become atrophied and feeble.

**Tendons**

Tendons are tough and robust tissues that connect muscles, bones, and joints, collectively referred to as tendons, including major tendons, minor tendons, and fascia.

Tendons serve to link joints, bones, and muscles, not only strengthening the stability of the joints but also playing a role in protecting and assisting muscle movements. Attaching to the joints, tendons contribute to joint flexibility, enabling smooth and coordinated movements.

The liver governs tendons. If there is insufficient blood in the liver and the blood fails to nourish the tendons, symptoms such as numbness in the limbs, difficulty in flexion and extension, stiffness in tendons and vessels, and tremors in the hands and feet may occur. When excessive pathogenic heat affects the liver's Yin and blood, symptoms of liver wind internal stirring may manifest, including limb convulsions, tremors in the hands and feet, tight closure of the jaw, and arching of the back.

**The Skeletal Bones**

The human body relies on the skeletal system as its backbone, with bones providing structural support to maintain a specific form and defend internal organs against external forces, thereby serving a protective function.

Bones also have the function of storing bone marrow, which nourishes the skeletal system. The growth, development, and brittleness of bones are all related to the abundance or deficiency of marrow.

Kidney essence plays a crucial role in promoting the growth, development, and repair of bones, hence the term "Kidneys govern bones." If there is a deficiency in kidney essence, resulting in empty marrow, it can lead to weak and feeble bones, and even developmental disorders in the skeletal system. Conditions such as delayed closure of fontanelles in children, weak and soft bones, and increased susceptibility to fractures in the elderly are associated with insufficient kidney essence.

Teeth are considered an extension of bones, as both teeth and bones originate from the same source. The growth and shedding of teeth are closely related to the abundance or decline of kidney essence.

## Main Functions of The Five Senses And Nine Orifices

The essence and energy of the five Zang organs are respectively connected to the seven orifices. Lung energy connects to the nose, and when the lungs are harmonious, the nose can perceive odors. Heart energy connects to the tongue, and when the heart is harmonious, the tongue can distinguish the five tastes. Liver energy connects to the eyes, and when the liver is harmonious, the eyes can differentiate between the five colors. Spleen energy connects to the mouth, and when the spleen is harmonious, the mouth can discern the five grains. Kidney energy connects to the ears, and when the kidneys are harmonious, the ears can hear the five sounds.

### Tongue

The tongue functions in sensory taste perception, aiding in chewing and swallowing food, and assisting in vocalization.

The heart opens into the tongue. When there is dysfunction in the heart's blood and vessel control, such as heart yang deficiency, the tongue may appear pale, fat, and tender. If there is insufficient heart blood, the tongue may appear pale. If there is an excess of heart fire, the tip of the tongue may be red. If there is stasis in the heart vessels, the tongue may appear purple with stasis points and patches. Abnormalities in the heart's governing of consciousness may manifest as a strong or rolled tongue, speech impediments, or loss of speech.

In tongue diagnosis, the specific areas correspond to different Zang organs: the tip of the tongue corresponds to the heart and lungs, the sides correspond to the liver and gallbladder (left liver, right gallbladder), the center corresponds to the spleen and stomach, and the root corresponds to the kidneys.

### Mouth

The oral cavity includes the lips, tongue, teeth, palate, pharynx, and more. The mouth is considered the exterior opening of the spleen, serving functions such as tasting and distinguishing the five flavors, secreting saliva, grinding food, aiding digestion, and facilitating speech.

The pharynx is an organ responsible for swallowing, breathing, and producing sound. It connects the oral cavity above to the nose and extends below to the lungs and stomach. It is also a vital point along the meridians. The front part of the pharynx, connected to the airway and vocal cords, is called the throat and is associated with the lungs. The posterior part connects to the esophagus, passing directly through the stomach, and is associated with the stomach.

The production of sound involves the coordinated action of various organs, including the lungs, vocal cords, tongue, lips, and uvula, all driven by the movement of lung Qi.

The pharynx serves as a shared organ for both digestion and respiration, with its main physiological function being the smooth passage of water and grains. The throat is associated with exhaling, connecting to the heavens, while the pharynx is associated with swallowing, connecting to the earth.

### Eyes

According to traditional Chinese medicine, the eye is mainly composed of five parts: the white sclera, black iris, pupil (or cornea), upper and lower eyelids, and inner and outer canthi. The white sclera is associated with the Qi wheel, the black iris with the Wind wheel, the pupil with the Water wheel, the inner and outer canthi with the Blood wheel, and the eyelids with the Flesh wheel. Therefore, the Blood wheel is related to the heart and small intestine, the Wind wheel to the liver and gallbladder, the Qi wheel to the lungs, large intestine, the Water wheel to the kidneys and bladder, and the Flesh wheel to the spleen and stomach.

The eyes have essential functions such as perceiving everything, examining details, distinguishing shapes, and identifying colors. They are formed by the innate essence and nurtured by acquired essence.

The eyes are considered the exterior reflection of the liver, and the liver opens into the eyes. Therefore, the condition of the liver often manifests in the eyes. For instance, if there is liver fire, the eyes may appear red and swollen. Conditions like liver wind internal stirring may result in strabismus or nystagmus. The visual function of the eyes depends not only on the overall nourishment of Qi and blood in the body's meridians but also on the moistening effect of the liver's Yin and blood. Therefore, many eye disorders are treated by considering both the overall condition and emphasizing the importance of liver health.

**Ears**

The ear is an organ responsible for hearing and equilibrium, and its physiological functions are closely related to the abundance or decline of essence and Qi in the kidneys.

The function of the ear relies on the nourishment of essence, marrow, Qi, and blood. When kidney essence is abundant and the marrow is well-nourished, hearing is sharp, and the power of discrimination is high. Conversely, when kidney essence is deficient and the marrow lacks nourishment, hearing loss, tinnitus, or deafness may occur.

In clinical practice, changes in hearing are often considered a sign to infer the strength or weakness of kidney Qi. As people age, the decline of essence and Qi in the kidneys gradually leads to a decrease in hearing ability.

The color of the face, hair, lips, nails, and hair can reflect the abundance or deficiency of Qi and blood in the five organs. The external manifestations of the five organs are seen in the face, hair, lips, nails, and hair: the radiance on the face corresponds to the heart, the luster of the hair to the lungs, the color of the lips to the spleen, the nails to the liver, and the hair to the kidneys.

When the heart functions well and the blood vessels are full, the complexion is rosy and glossy. If there is insufficient heart Qi or blood, the complexion becomes pale without radiance.

If the lung Qi is imbalanced and cannot circulate Qi and body fluids to nourish the hair, the hair may become dull and lifeless.

When the spleen loses its healthy function, and there is deficiency in Qi and blood, the lips may appear pale and lack radiance, or even become withered and yellow. Cracking or ulceration of the lips may indicate heat accumulation in the spleen and stomach, while a dark color around the lips and lip curling, unable to cover the teeth, are signs of severe spleen Qi deficiency.

When the liver blood is sufficient, the nails are strong, resilient, and bright. If there is insufficient liver blood, the nails may become soft, thin, and discolored, or even deformed or brittle.

Since hair is an external manifestation of kidney function, the growth, shedding, moisture, and withering of hair are closely related to kidney essence.

## Life Activities of the Human Body And Regulation of the Five Organs

Let's talk about the life activities of the human body and the regulation of the five organs.

The basic life activities of the human body mainly refer to activities such as consciousness, respiratory movement, digestion and absorption, blood circulation, water metabolism, growth, and reproduction. In a healthy state, these manifest as the normal physiological functions of the human body, while in a pathological state, they reflect abnormal life phenomena in the diseased organism.

The human body is an organic and unified system centered around the five organs. Qi and blood constitute the material basis of the life activities of the human body. The functions of the organs coordinate and balance, yin and yang harmonize, and qi and blood flow smoothly, maintaining the unity of the body with its environment, ensuring the normal life activities of the human body.

**Consciousness and Movements of the Mind**

The heart houses the spirit, which means that the heart governs and dominates activities such as consciousness, thoughts, and emotions. The four spirits of the soul, corporeal soul, intention, and will, as well as the five emotions of joy, anger, thought, worry, and fear, are all under the control of the heart spirit.

The lungs house the corporeal soul, which belongs to the instinctive sensations and actions of the human body, i.e., unconscious activities. Examples include the auditory perception of the ears, visual perception of the eyes, sensory perceptions of cold, heat, pain, and itching in the skin, as well as movements of the trunk and limbs, newborns' sucking and crying, etc., all fall under the domain of the corporeal soul. The corporeal soul is innate, acquired from birth, and is stored in the lungs. Therefore, when lung qi is vigorous, the body is healthy, and the corporeal soul is complete. A complete corporeal soul results in heightened sensitivity, keen hearing, clear vision, and correct and coordinated movements.

The liver houses the "hun" (similar to spirit) referring to the thought and conscious activities that can respond quickly to the activities of the heart spirit, including dreaming. The liver governs the dispersion and storage of blood. When liver qi flows smoothly and blood is abundant, the "hun" can follow the spirit, and its functions can be normally expressed. If the liver fails to disperse or if there is insufficient liver blood, the "hun" cannot follow the spirit, leading to symptoms such as confusion, vivid dreams, and restless sleep. Closely associated with the cloudy "hun" (◇), there is the white-cloudy "po"◇◇◇. The "hun" is associated with yang, while the "po" is associated with yin.

The spleen houses the intention, where thoughts involve selecting and retaining knowledge acquired from the external world, forming impressions that become memories. When the spleen's qi is robust, the transformation of nutrients is sufficient, and the qi and blood are abundant, the marrow is nourished, resulting in clear thinking, rich thoughts, and strong memory.

The kidneys house the will. A steadfast will means that the intention is determined, unwavering, and committed to practical actions in the future. Kidney essence produces marrow, which ascends to the brain. When the marrow is abundant, the spirit is vigorous, and the conscious activities of the will are normal.

In Traditional Chinese Medicine, there are distinctions between the concepts of "Five Emotions (◇)" and "Seven Emotional Expressions (◇)." The human emotional states are categorized into five emotions, namely anger, joy, thought, worry, and grief: the liver "expresses anger," the heart "expresses joy," the spleen "expresses thought," the lungs "expresses worry," and the kidneys "express fear," hence referred to as the Five Emotions.

The seven emotional expressions are joy, anger, worry, thought, grief, fear, and surprise.

**Circulation of Blood**

Traditional Chinese Medicine believes that blood is one of the fundamental substances constituting the human body and essential for maintaining life activities. It plays a crucial role in nourishing and moisturizing the body. Blood circulates within the vessels, reaching the internal organs and extending to the skin, muscles, tendons, and bones, providing nourishment and moisture to various organs and tissues throughout the body.

The normal circulation of blood relies on the propelling, warming, and consolidating functions of qi (vital energy). The direction of blood circulation includes two aspects: centrifugal (leaving the heart) and centripetal (returning to the heart). Centrifugal circulation refers to the blood leaving the heart, traveling through the meridians to the network vessels, branching repeatedly, and gradually narrowing into smaller vessels, ultimately reaching all tissues and organs throughout the body. Centripetal circulation involves blood, after being utilized by various tissues and organs, carrying waste products through the capillaries to the network vessels, gradually converging into the meridians, and finally returning to the heart.

The heart governs the blood vessels, serving as the fundamental force for blood circulation. The normal movement of blood throughout the body relies on the propelling force of heart qi, ensuring its proper distribution.

**Respiration Process**

The process of respiration refers to the exchange of gases where the human body inhales fresh air from the natural environment and exhales stale air, involving the expulsion of waste gases and the intake of fresh air.

During the inhalation process, the lungs, through the descending action, draw in fresh air from the natural environment either through the nasal or oral cavities. The air then travels through the throat, trachea, and other respiratory passages before entering the lungs. The fresh air descends along the meridians to the kidneys, where it is absorbed and stored, providing a place for the air to return to. Simultaneously, this process continuously nourishes the kidney qi.

In the exhalation process, the body produces stale air during metabolic activities. The majority of this stale air ascends through the meridians to the heart and lungs. Under the action of the lungs, it then travels through the respiratory passages such as the trachea, throat, and nose before being expelled from the body. Some portion of the stale air is also excreted through the opening and closing of the pores in the skin.

The lungs govern the qi, and the kidneys are the root of qi. The lungs control the exhalation of qi, while the kidneys govern the inhalation of qi. The interaction of yin and yang is essential for harmonious breathing. The liver governs the dispersion and regulates the smooth flow of qi. The liver, being a solid organ, governs the dispersion, while the lungs, being a delicate organ, control the descending action. The liver ascends from the left, and the lungs descend from the right. When the ascending and descending actions are appropriate, the flow of qi is smooth. The spleen governs transformation, and the essence of food and drink ascends from the spleen. It combines with the respiratory qi of the lungs to generate ancestral qi. Ancestral qi travels through the respiratory passages, governs respiration, and permeates the heart meridian to circulate qi and blood.

**Digestion and Absorption**

Digestion and absorption are two essential processes in the metabolism of dietary substances. Through the movement of the digestive organs and the action of digestive fluids, food is separated into clear and turbid components, transformed into refined nutrients that can be absorbed and utilized. On the basis of thorough digestion, the refined substances are absorbed and then transported to the heart and lungs. Digestion and absorption are closely connected, mutually supportive, and coordinated processes.

The process of digestion and absorption of dietary substances is closely related to the physiological activities of the five Zang organs (heart, liver, spleen, lungs, kidneys) and six Fu organs (gallbladder, stomach, small intestine, large intestine, bladder, triple burner). The coordination of functions among these organs, including the spleen, stomach, small intestine, large intestine, liver, gallbladder, and pancreas, is crucial in the digestive and absorptive processes. The relationship between the spleen, small intestine, and stomach is particularly intimate. Therefore, it is said that the spleen and stomach are the foundation of acquired constitution, the source of the transformation of qi and blood.

### Flow of Body Fluids

Body fluids originate from diet and are generated through digestion and absorption, primarily involving the stomach, spleen, and small and large intestines. The metabolic process of body fluids is centered around the spleen, lungs, and kidneys.

After the generation of body fluids, the spleen, through its ascending and clarifying functions, transports them upward to the heart and lungs. Simultaneously, a portion of the unabsorbed body fluids, along with food residues, descends to the large intestine and is expelled from the body through feces.

The lungs receive a significant amount of body fluids from the spleen and, through their disseminating and descending functions, distribute them throughout the body. Some of the body fluids, under the influence of the lungs' disseminating function, circulate on the body surface, reaching the extremities and openings, nourishing muscles, moisturizing the skin, and eliminating metabolic waste and residual moisture. Through the evaporation facilitated by yang qi, they transform into sweat and are expelled through sweat pores. Another portion of body fluids, influenced by the lungs' descending function and propelled by the heart's energy, circulates internally along the meridians with the nutrient qi, nourishing the internal organs, permeating the bones and brain marrow. After being utilized by the body's tissues and organs, they gather in the kidneys. Additionally, a small amount of water vapor is expelled during the lung's exhalation movement.

The kidneys are the primary organ governing water, and the fluids gathered in the kidneys undergo a process of gasification, resulting in the separation of clear and turbid components. The clear component, through the vaporization and gasification of the kidney's yang qi, ascends back to the lungs. From there, it is dispersed throughout the body by the heart and lungs, maintaining the normal fluid balance within the body. The turbid component, driven by the warming and transforming action of the kidney's yang qi, continuously transforms into urine and is directed downward to the bladder. When the urine accumulates to a certain level in the bladder, a sense of urgency arises, prompting timely voluntary expulsion through the urethra.

Body fluids include all normal and abnormal fluids in the human body. It includes the normal body fluids and secretions of various organs and tissues, such as gastric fluid, intestinal fluid, saliva, synovial fluid, etc. It also encompasses metabolic by-products such as urine, sweat, tears, etc. The functions of body fluids mainly involve moisturizing and nourishing, generating blood, regulating yin and yang, and eliminating waste products.

Body fluids originate from diet, generated through the digestion and absorption of water and nutrients in the diet by the spleen, stomach, small intestine, and large intestine.

The distribution of body fluids relies on the comprehensive functions of various organs, including the spleen, lungs, kidneys, liver, heart, and triple burner.

Insufficient generation or excessive loss of body fluids can lead to damage to the body fluids, resulting in dryness. In severe cases, it may lead to deficiency of yin fluids and even loss of yin, requiring treatment to nourish fluids, supplement yin fluids, and restrain fluids to save yin. When body fluids stagnate, it can manifest as dampness, phlegm, edema, and the treatment approach should involve sweating, dampness transformation, diuresis, water elimination, and phlegm expulsion.

The Five Liquids are produced by the five Zang organs: sweat by the heart, nasal fluids by the lungs, tears by the liver, salivary fluid by the spleen, and saliva by the kidneys. Sweat is considered the fluid of the heart, nasal fluids of the lungs, tears of the liver, salivary fluid of the spleen, and saliva of the kidneys.

Qi, blood, body fluids, essence, and other substances are fundamental components of the human body and essential for maintaining life activities. They are continuously replenished by the spleen and stomach transforming water and grains. Under the guidance of organ functions and the dominion of the spirit, these substances permeate, promote, and transform each other in a dynamic interplay.

# Chapter 4

# Overview of the Meridian and Collateral System

The theory of meridians and collaterals is the study of the composition, circulation, physiological functions, pathological changes, and the interrelationships with organs, qi, and blood of the human meridian system. It is a crucial part of traditional Chinese medicine (TCM) theory and serves as the theoretical core of acupuncture and massage.

"Meridians" is a collective term for "jing" (◇) and "luo" (◇). "Jing," also known as meridians, implies a pathway. Meridians traverse the body vertically, connecting the internal and external, forming the main trunk of the meridian system. "Luo," also known as collateral vessels, implies a network. Collateral vessels are branches that diverge from the meridians and are finer in comparison. They crisscross and network throughout the body, reaching every part.

The human body is composed of the five Zang organs, six Fu organs, four limbs, hundreds of bones, five sensory organs, nine orifices, skin, muscles, blood vessels, and bones. Although they have different physiological functions, they collectively engage in organic activities, maintaining coordination and unity between the internal and external, upper and lower aspects of the body, forming an organic whole. This organic coordination and interconnection mainly rely on the communication and connection provided by meridians.

Due to the intricate interweaving of the twelve meridians and their branches, their vertical and horizontal crossings, and their connections from the interior to the exterior, the meridians interconnect with each other, link to the Zang-Fu organs, and connect the extraordinary vessels. The extraordinary vessels link and communicate with the twelve regular meridians. The twelve meridians and their associated tendons, muscles, and skin form a closely connected and coordinated unity between the internal organs and tissues, creating a well-coordinated and unified whole in terms of the interior and exterior, upper and lower aspects of the body.

**The Twelve Meridians**

There are twelve primary meridians, which are the Hand and Foot Three Yin and Three Yang meridians, forming four groups collectively referred to as the twelve meridians. Their names are as follows: Hand Taiyin Lung Meridian, Hand Jueyin Pericardium Meridian, Hand Shaoyin Heart Meridian, Hand Yangming Large Intestine Meridian, Hand Shaoyang San Jiao Meridian, Hand Taiyang Small Intestine Meridian, Foot Taiyin Spleen Meridian, Foot Jueyin Liver Meridian, Foot Shaoyin Kidney Meridian, Foot Yangming Stomach Meridian, Foot Shaoyang Gallbladder Meridian, and Foot Taiyang Bladder Meridian.

**The twelve associated meridians** represent the twelve main pathways that run through the body, connecting the limbs, internal organs, and emerging superficially at the neck. The Yang meridians branch out from their original paths, coursing through the body, reaching the head and face, and then returning to their primary meridian. On the other hand, the Yin meridians also branch out from their primary paths, travel through the body, reach the head and face, and combine with their corresponding Yang meridian, forming a relationship known as the exterior and interior.

**The twelve tendino-muscular meridians** connect and link all the bones, network throughout the body, and play a role in governing joint movements.

The eight extraordinary vessels are the Governing Vessel (Du Mai), Conception Vessel (Ren Mai), Thrusting Vessel (Chong Mai), Girdle Vessel (Dai Mai), Yin Linking Vessel (Yin Wei Mai), Yang Linking Vessel (Yang Wei Mai), Yin Motility Vessel (Yin Qiao Mai), and Yang Motility Vessel (Yang Qiao Mai). The eight extraordinary vessels have the functions of regulating, connecting, and harmonizing the abundance and decline of qi and blood throughout the entire body.

The Three Yin of the Hand ascend from the chest to the hand; the Three Yang of the Hand ascend from the hand to the head; the Three Yang of the Foot ascend from the head to the foot; the Three Yin of the Foot ascend from the foot to the abdomen. This is the directional pattern of the twelve meridians.

The Yin meridians connect with the Yang meridians at the junctions of the limbs. The Three Yang of the Hand and Foot intersect in the head and face. The Yin meridians intersect in the chest and abdomen.

In the circulation of the twelve meridians, those related to the six Zang organs (plus the Pericardium) are termed Yin meridians, and they mostly circulate along the inner sides of the limbs and the chest and abdomen. Those related to the six Fu organs are termed Yang meridians, and they mostly circulate along the outer sides of the limbs and the head, face, and trunk.

The distribution characteristics of the twelve meridians in the head and face are as follows: Hand and Foot Yangming meridians distribute in the forehead area; Hand Taiyang meridian distributes in the cheek area; Hand and Foot Shaoyang meridians distribute in the ear and temple area; Foot Taiyang meridian distributes in the top of the head and occipital region. Additionally, the Foot Jueyin meridian also courses to the top.

The distribution pattern of the twelve meridians in the head and face is as follows: Yangming is in the front, Shaoyang is on the side, and Taiyang is in the back.

The general distribution pattern of the twelve meridians in the trunk is as follows: The Foot Three Yin and Foot Yangming meridians distribute in the chest and abdomen; the Hand Three Yang and Foot Taiyang meridians distribute in the shoulders, scapulae, back, and waist; the Hand Three Yin, Foot Shaoyang, and Foot Jueyin meridians distribute in the axillary region, flanks, and lateral abdominal areas.

The flow of the twelve meridians begins with the Hand Taiyin Lung Meridian, then proceeds sequentially to the Foot Jueyin Liver Meridian, and finally returns to the Hand Taiyin Lung Meridian. This forms a complete circulation system of the twelve meridians, creating a "circulation without end" where Yin and Yang mutually penetrate.

The Yellow Emperor's Internal Classic states: "Meridians are the pathways for determining life and death, addressing myriad diseases, regulating deficiencies and excesses; they must not be blocked." "Meridians serve to circulate blood and qi, nourish Yin and Yang, moisten tendons and bones, and facilitate joint movement."

The meridians crisscross and interconnect, spreading throughout the entire body, linking the internal and external, organs, limbs, and sensory orifices, forming an organic whole. In the vital activities of the human body, meridians play a highly significant physiological role.

In clinical practice, symptoms manifested by diseases, combined with the locations of meridian circulation and their connection to internal organs, can be used as the basis for diagnosing illnesses. For example, pain on both sides of the ribcage is often related to liver and gallbladder diseases, while lower abdominal pain may indicate lung pathology. Similarly, in cases of headaches, pain in the frontal region is often associated with the Yangming meridian, pain on both sides with the Shaoyang meridian, pain at the back of the head and neck with the Taiyang meridian, and pain at the crown with the Jueyin meridian. The differentiation of the Six Meridians in the Treatise on Cold Damage is also a diagnostic system developed based on meridian theory.

Acupuncture and massage therapy primarily target specific meridians or organs affected by pathology. Acupoints are selected in nearby or distant areas along the meridian pathways to adjust the functional activities of meridian qi and blood. Through acupuncture or massage, the goal is to achieve therapeutic effects by harmonizing the functions of the meridians and promoting overall balance.

# Chapter 5

## Causes of Diseases

The etiology refers to specific factors that can disrupt the dynamic balance of the human body, leading to the occurrence of diseases. Pathogenic factors, when acting on the human body, disrupt the physiological state of the organism, causing certain imbalances, disturbances, or impairments in morphology, function, and metabolism. In traditional Chinese medicine, the causes of diseases are believed to include the Six Exogenous Pathogenic Factors (Six Evils), epidemic toxins, Seven Emotions, diet, overexertion, external injuries, as well as phlegm, dampness, stasis, and other factors.

However, whether it's the invasion of external Six Evils, the internal disturbances caused by Seven Emotions, dietary imbalances, or excessive exertion, they will not lead to illness as long as the body's righteous qi is strong, and physiological functions are normal. Disease occurs only when the righteous qi is weakened, and the body's functional activities cannot adapt to changes in various factors, making them pathogenic factors that trigger illness.

During the development of a disease, causes and results interact and constrain each other. Under certain conditions, the relationship between cause and effect can be mutually transformed. In one pathological stage, it may be the result of pathology, while in another stage, it could become a cause of disease. For example, phlegm and blood stasis are pathological products formed due to the imbalance of organ qi and blood functions. However, once these pathological products are formed, they can become new causes, leading to other pathological changes and the manifestation of various symptoms and signs.

Based on the pathogenesis and formation process of diseases, causes are generally categorized as exogenous causes, endogenous causes, causes formed by pathological products, and other causes.

## External Pathogenic Factors

Let's discuss the external pathogenic factors known as the "Six Qi" and "Six Evils."

The "Six Qi" refers to six normal climatic conditions in the natural environment: wind, cold, heat, dampness, dryness, and fire.

The "Six Evils" refer to six types of pathogenic factors causing external diseases: wind, cold, heat, dampness, dryness, and fire.

When the Six Evils affect the human body, penetrating from the surface to the interior and harming the organs, they can easily lead to the internal generation of the "Five Evils." The Five Evils manifest as disturbances in the functions of the organs and viscera, making the body susceptible to the invasion of the Six Evils once again. This interplay between external pathogenic factors and internal imbalances contributes to the progression of diseases.

### Wind Evil

The nature and pathogenic characteristics of Wind Evil: Wind has a light and ascending nature, easily causing multiple changes. When Wind dominates, it induces movement and becomes the origin of various illnesses. This is the fundamental characteristic of the Wind Evil.

Wind, being a yang pathogenic factor, has a light and upward-scattering nature, manifesting characteristics of ascending, rising, and spreading outward. Therefore, when Wind Evil causes diseases, it tends to harm the upper part of the body and frequently affects the muscles, skin, and the lumbar region, which are considered as yang locations. The lungs, as the "◇◇" (flowering canopy) among the five viscera and six bowels, can be affected by Wind Evil, leading to symptoms such as nasal congestion, runny nose, itchy throat, and cough. When Wind Evil disturbs the head and face, symptoms may include dizziness, headache, strong pain in the head and neck, facial muscle paralysis, and deviation of the mouth and eyes.

The pathogenic influence of Wind Evil is characterized by instability and constant movement. This often manifests as symptoms like dizziness, tremors, convulsions in the limbs, and opisthotonus.

As Wind is associated with the Wood element and connected to the Liver, the pathogenic effect of Wind Evil on the Liver can result in symptoms such as epigastric pain, abdominal distension, bowel rumbling, vomiting, and diarrhea.

**Cold Evil**

Nature and pathogenic characteristics of Cold Evil: Cold Evil is characterized by coldness, coagulation, and contraction.

Cold Evil directly invades the interior, causing symptoms such as vomiting and diarrhea with clear, watery substances and cold pain in the epigastrium if it affects the Spleen and Stomach. When the Lungs and Spleen are affected by cold, it can manifest as coughing, rapid breathing, thin or edematous phlegm. Cold damage to the Spleen and Kidneys may result in symptoms such as aversion to cold, cold limbs, cold and painful lower back, clear and loose urine, and abdominal edema. If there is a deficiency of Heart and Kidney Yang, symptoms may include aversion to cold, curling up, cold extremities, clear and copious diarrhea, mental fatigue, and a faint pulse.

Cold Evil invades the muscles and surfaces, causing severe pain in the head, body, and joints. If Cold Evil directly impacts the interior and obstructs the flow of Qi, it can lead to cold pain or twisting pain in the chest, epigastrium, and abdomen.

When Cold Evil affects the meridians and joints, it causes contraction and stiffness in the tendons and vessels, resulting in spasms, difficulty in flexion and extension, or cold-induced loss of consciousness.

**Heat Evil**

Nature and pathogenic characteristics of Heat Evil: Heat Evil is the transformation of Fire, primarily characterized by ascending and dispersing, often accompanied by dampness.

When Heat Evil harms the body, it typically manifests a series of symptoms associated with Yang and heat, such as high fever, restlessness, facial flushing, irritability, and a strong and large pulse. If excessive sweating injures body fluids, it may lead to symptoms such as thirst with a preference for drinking, dry lips and tongue, and scanty dark urine. In severe cases, it can cause Qi deficiency, shortness of breath, fatigue, sudden fainting, and heatstroke with loss of consciousness.

In hot and humid weather, the prevalence of dampness is common. The clinical features, in addition to symptoms of heat such as fever and thirst, often include fatigue in the limbs, chest tightness, nausea, and loose or unsatisfactory stools.

**Factor of Dampness**

Nature and pathogenic characteristics of Dampness: Dampness is considered a Yin pathogen that obstructs the flow of Qi, easily injuring Yang Qi. Its nature is heavy, turbid, sticky, and tends to descend.

When Dampness invades the human body, it tends to afflict the Spleen, leading to weakened Spleen Yang, impaired transformation and transportation functions, and the accumulation of water-dampness, resulting in symptoms such as diarrhea, edema, and reduced urine output.

The clinical manifestations of illness caused by Dampness have a characteristic heaviness, such as a feeling of heaviness and fatigue in the head and body, and a sensation of soreness and heaviness in the limbs. If Dampness affects the skin or joints, it can lead to symptoms such as a heavy or foggy feeling in the head, akin to being wrapped or bound; or joint pain and stiffness when Dampness stagnates in the meridians and joints. The turbid and sticky nature of Dampness can result in symptoms like greasy facial complexion, excessive tears, loose or sticky stools with mucus or blood in the case of Dampness affecting the Large Intestine, and cloudy or abundant vaginal discharge in women. Dampness soaking the skin can lead to conditions such as ulcers, eczema, and the formation of turbid or purulent fluids.

**Factor of Dryness**

The nature and pathogenic characteristics of Dryness: Dryness leads to dryness, and it easily injures the Lungs, which is a fundamental characteristic of Dryness as a pathogen.

When Dryness causes harm, it most easily consumes the body's fluids, resulting in various symptoms and signs of dryness, such as dry and cracked skin, dry nose and throat, chapped lips, dry and lusterless hair, scanty urination, and dry stools.

Dryness invading the Lungs damages the Lung fluids, impairing their function of dispersing and descending, thereby leading to symptoms like dry cough with little or difficult-to-expectorate phlegm, or phlegm mixed with blood, as well as wheezing and chest pain.

**The Factor of Heat**

The nature and pathogenic characteristics of Heat: Heat pathogen exhibits characteristics of scorching, inflammation, consuming Qi and injuring fluids, and generating Wind and agitating Blood.

When the Heat pathogen causes disease, the manifestation of heat is prominent, characterized by fever and rapid pulse. For instance, if Heart Heat flares up, symptoms may include a red and painful tongue tip, oral ulcers, and the formation of sores; if Liver Heat flares up, symptoms may include severe headache, red and swollen eyes, and eye pain; when Stomach Heat is excessive, symptoms may involve swollen and painful gums, as well as gum bleeding.

When Wind and Heat mutually exacerbate, symptoms become urgent and severe, clinically presenting as high fever, delirium, convulsions, neck stiffness, opisthotonus, and upward deviation of the eyes.

The Heat pathogen, in its scorching nature, damages blood vessels, accelerates blood circulation, and may lead to various types of bleeding, such as hematemesis, epistaxis, hematochezia, hematuria, as well as skin rashes. Heat toxins are common causes of ulcers and sores, with local manifestations of redness, swelling, and heat.

### The Qi of Epidemic Pathogens

The qi of epidemic pathogens refers to a highly contagious pathogenic factor. Epidemic qi spreads through the air and contact. Unlike the Six External Pathogens, it is not a pathogenic factor formed by changes in climate but rather a type of pathogenic microorganism that cannot be directly observed by human senses. Epidemic qi enters the body through various pathways, such as the mouth and nose, making it an external pathogenic factor.

Unlike warm diseases, which are a general term for various acute febrile diseases caused by external pathogens, warm diseases lack contagiousness and epidemicity. Epidemic pathogens are characterized by strong contagiousness, wide prevalence, and high mortality rates.

### Factors of Internal Damages

### Seven Emotional Expressions

Emotional activities such as joy, anger, worry, contemplation, grief, fear, and surprise can lead to the occurrence of various diseases and have a significant impact on the development of illnesses. These emotions can either promote improvement or deterioration of the patient's condition.

The basic rules regarding the impact of the Seven Emotions on the internal organs are as follows: Joy is associated with the Heart; excessive joy can harm the Heart. Anger is associated with the Liver; excessive anger can harm the Liver. Contemplation is associated with the Spleen; excessive contemplation can harm the Spleen. Grief and worry are associated with the Lungs; excessive grief and worry can harm the Lungs. Fear is associated with the Kidneys; excessive fear can harm the Kidneys.

Emotional imbalances primarily affect the Heart, Liver, and Spleen, leading to disruptions in the balance of Qi and blood. For instance, excessive joy may damage the Heart, leading to symptoms such as restlessness, insomnia, irritability, anxiety, confusion, and even abnormal mental states like unpredictable laughter, tears, constant talking, and manic behavior. Unresolved anger can harm the Liver, affecting its regulatory functions and resulting in symptoms like rib-side distension and pain, emotional irritability, frequent sighing, a sensation of a lump in the throat, or irregular menstruation and abdominal masses due to Qi stagnation and blood stasis. Excessive worry may harm the Spleen, causing symptoms such as loss of appetite and abdominal distension.

It is crucial to recognize the impact of emotions on health, as emotional imbalances can contribute to the development and progression of various health issues.

**Improper Dietary Habits**

Improper dietary habits, such as excessive eating, unclean or biased food preferences, can lead to the occurrence of diseases and are one of the main factors contributing to internal injuries.

Overindulgence in food and drink, surpassing the digestive and absorptive capacities of the Spleen and Stomach, can result in food stagnation. Symptoms of food-induced Spleen and Stomach disorders may include abdominal distension, acid regurgitation, aversion to food, and vomiting.

Prolonged overeating can obstruct the circulation of Qi and blood in the gastrointestinal meridians, leading to diarrhea, rectal bleeding, hemorrhoids, and other issues. Excessive consumption of fatty and sweet foods may generate internal heat, potentially causing conditions like abscesses and ulcers.

Consuming overly spicy, warm, or drying foods can accumulate heat in the gastrointestinal tract, resulting in symptoms such as thirst, abdominal fullness, pain, and constipation, or even contributing to the development of hemorrhoids.

Excessive food intake can lead to accumulation and excess; excessive thirst may lead to the accumulation of dampness and the generation of phlegm. For example, an excessive preference for fermented foods may lead to the accumulation of water and edema, while an excessive preference for melons, fruits, milk, and butter can generate internal dampness, leading to swelling, fullness, and diarrhea.

Insufficient food intake can result in a lack of nutritional sources, leading to reduced Qi and blood. Insufficient Qi and blood can manifest as emaciation, weakened vital energy, and lowered resistance to illnesses.

Excessive consumption of salty foods may cause blood stasis and a loss of luster in the complexion. Overindulgence in bitter foods may result in dry skin and hair loss. Consuming an excess of pungent foods may cause stiffness in the tendons and nails becoming dry and withered. Consuming too much sour food can lead to thickened and wrinkled skin, thin and dry lips. Finally, consuming an excess of sweet foods may cause bone pain and hair loss.

**Excessive Physical Labor or Indulgence**

Excessive physical labor can damage internal organ functions, leading to deficiency in organ Qi. Symptoms may include weakness, fatigue, lethargy, reluctance to speak, mental exhaustion, and emaciation.

Overexertion of the mind can deplete heart blood, impair spleen Qi, resulting in symptoms such as palpitations, forgetfulness, insomnia, vivid dreams, poor appetite, abdominal bloating, and loose stools. In severe cases, excessive mental strain can deplete Qi and damage blood, weakening the functions of organs, causing deficiency in vital energy, and even leading to chronic illnesses due to accumulated fatigue.

Excessive sexual activity refers to immoderate sexual behavior. While normal sexual activity generally does not harm the body, excessive sexual activity can deplete kidney essence, leading to symptoms such as sore and weak lower back and knees, dizziness, tinnitus, mental fatigue, or in men, nocturnal emissions, premature ejaculation, decreased sexual function, and even impotence.

Excessive indulgence refers to a lifestyle of excessive comfort without adequate physical activity. This sedentary lifestyle disrupts the smooth circulation of Qi and blood, makes tendons and bones fragile, causes stagnation in the spleen and stomach, and results in physical weakness, fatigue, or obesity with associated symptoms like palpitations, shortness of breath, and excessive sweating. It can also lead to the development of other diseases.

## Pathological Factors

Phlegm-dampness, blood stasis, and calculi are pathological products formed during the course of diseases. When they linger in the body without being eliminated, they can become new pathogenic factors.

### Phlegm-dampness

Phlegm-dampness manifests different symptoms in various parts of the body, showing diverse clinical presentations. These manifestations can be summarized as the eight major symptoms: cough, wheezing, palpitations, dizziness, nausea, fullness, swelling, and pain.

When phlegm-dampness flows along the meridians, it can easily cause blockages in the meridians, disrupting the smooth circulation of Qi and blood. This may result in symptoms such as numbness in the limbs, limited range of motion, or even hemiplegia. If it accumulates locally, it can lead to the formation of lymph node tuberculosis in the neck, jaw, and limbs, abscesses in muscles, tendons, and bones, as well as suppuration in deep tissues.

### Blood Stasis

After the formation of blood stasis, not only does it lose the nourishing effect of normal blood, but it also adversely affects the circulation of blood throughout the body or in specific areas. This can lead to pain, bleeding, blockage of meridians, accumulation of blood stasis in organs, and adverse consequences such as "when blood stasis persists, new blood cannot be generated."

In addition, commonly observed symptoms include dark complexion, nail abnormalities, skin purpura, and psychological and neurological symptoms (such as forgetfulness, restlessness, and coma).

Blood stasis can cause a wide range of diseases, and its clinical manifestations vary depending on the location of stasis and the reasons for the formation of blood stasis. Blood stasis in the heart may manifest as palpitations, chest tightness, chest pain, and bluish lips and nails. Blood stasis in the lungs may lead to chest pain and coughing up blood. If blood stasis occurs in the stomach and intestines, vomiting blood and black, tarry stools may result. Liver blood stasis may cause pain and masses in the hypochondrium. Blood stasis attacking the heart can lead to madness. Blood stasis in the uterus can cause lower abdominal pain, irregular menstruation, painful periods, amenorrhea, and clots in the menstrual blood, or excessive bleeding. In the limbs, blood stasis can result in ulceration, and in localized areas of the skin and muscles, there may be swelling, pain, and bluish discoloration.

**Formation of Stones**

Improper diet, emotional disturbances, inappropriate medication, and the retention of drugs in the body can lead to the dysfunction of organs, inducing the formation of stones. External factors such as the six climatic evils and excessive comfort can also result in unfavorable Qi circulation, the generation of damp-heat, and the formation of stones. Additionally, the occurrence of stones is related to factors such as age, gender, constitution, and lifestyle habits.

When stones accumulate and obstruct the Qi circulation, affecting the flow of Qi and blood, they can damage the organs. This blockage of organ Qi circulation leads to pain, which is a fundamental characteristic. Stones are more likely to form in organs such as the gallbladder, stomach, liver, kidneys, and bladder.

**Other Pathogenic Factors**

External injury refers to factors that cause damage to the skin, muscles, tendons, and bones due to external forces such as impact, falls, cuts from sharp objects, as well as bites or burns from insects and animals.

Injuries from insects and animals include bites from poisonous snakes, attacks by wild animals, and bites from rabid dogs, among others. Mild cases may result in local swelling, pain, and bleeding, while severe cases can lead to internal organ damage, excessive bleeding, or even death if toxic substances penetrate internally.

Parasites residing within the human body not only consume the body's nutrients, such as Qi, blood, and bodily fluids, but also damage the physiological functions of organs, leading to the occurrence of diseases.

Diseases caused by prenatal factors are referred to as prenatal syndromes or prenatal diseases. Examples of prenatal disorders include prenatal cold, prenatal heat, excessive fetal fat, weak fetus, fetal toxins, fontanelle abnormalities, and the five soft spots, all falling within the scope of prenatal illnesses.

# Chapter 6

## Pathogenesis in TCM Terms

The mechanism of disease occurrence, development, and changes reveals the essential characteristics and basic laws of the onset, progression, changes, and outcomes of diseases.

In traditional Chinese medicine, it is believed that in the process of disease occurrence and development, the invasion of pathogenic factors (evil qi) and the weakening of righteous qi are indispensable factors. The struggle between pathogenic qi and righteous qi, as well as the contrast in their strengths, often influences the direction and outcome of the disease.

When righteous qi is strong and can resist pathogenic factors, the disease does not manifest. However, if righteous qi is weak and unable to withstand the invasion of pathogenic factors, the disease occurs.

After the invasion of pathogenic factors, the body's righteous qi can rise to resist them. However, before the pathogenic factors are completely expelled, physiological functions have already been disrupted, leading to corresponding clinical symptoms, indicating the formation of a certain type of disease. Nevertheless, individuals with weakened constitutions often require the invasion of pathogenic factors to a certain depth before the righteous qi can be activated. Consequently, their illnesses tend to be more severe, with a deeper pathological location.

Once pathogenic factors invade the human body, the specific location of the illness depends on the strength or weakness of the righteous qi in various parts of the body. For example, if the qi in the organs is deficient, the disease manifests in the organs; if the qi in the viscera is insufficient, the disease manifests in the viscera; and if the qi in the meridians is inadequate, the disease manifests along the meridians.

Traditional Chinese medicine holds that after the invasion of pathogenic factors, these factors may remain in the body without immediate symptoms. Due to various factors such as imbalances in diet, daily routines, or emotional fluctuations, the normal circulation of qi and blood in the body is disrupted. This leads to a decline in the body's immune function, allowing pathogenic factors to take advantage, engaging in a struggle with righteous qi and causing the onset of disease. Therefore, in clinical practice, certain diseases are often observed to fluctuate with the rise and fall of righteous qi, manifesting periods of exacerbation, improvement, or recurrence. Consequently, while pathogenic factors can contribute to illness, they typically cause harm and lead to disease under conditions of weakened righteous qi.

The interaction between righteous qi and pathogenic factors, as well as their struggle, is influenced by various factors both within and outside the body. The external environment of the body includes natural and social environments, mainly related to the nature and quantity of pathogenic factors. The internal environment comprises constitutional factors, mental state, genetic factors, etc., and is closely related to the body's righteous qi.

Human constitution exhibits a bias towards yin or yang. After the invasion of external pathogenic factors, the resulting illness is individualized, with the nature and manifestations of the disease changing accordingly.

After being exposed to external pathogenic factors, due to the individual characteristics of one's constitution, there are often varied changes in the pathological nature of the illness. For instance, when encountering the pathogenic influence of wind-cold, individuals with a yang-heat constitution tend to transform it into yang-heat, while those with a yin-cold constitution are more prone to transforming it into yin-cold.

If there is an inherent deficiency in one's constitution, coupled with constitutional weakness and emotional imbalances, the righteous qi weakens, the body's resistance declines, and pathogenic factors are more likely to invade and cause illness.

The types of disease onset generally include sudden onset, latent onset, gradual onset, intermittent onset, consecutive onset, combined and concurrent diseases, relapses, etc.

Invasions by the Six Pathogenic Factors, intense emotional fluctuations, diseases caused by epidemic factors, poisoning, accidental injuries, etc., can lead to immediate and acute manifestations, characterized by sudden and rapid onset.

After certain pathogenic factors enter the human body, they may not immediately cause illness but instead remain latent within. After a period of time or under certain triggering factors, the illness may then manifest. Examples of such conditions include tetanus, rabies, etc.

Regarding diseases caused by external factors, cold and damp pathogenic influences, being yin in nature, tend to be stagnant, viscous, and heavy, often resulting in a slow onset of disease.

Secondary diseases inevitably have the primary disease as a prerequisite. For instance, complications such as flank pain and jaundice arising from viral hepatitis may develop if not properly treated or if the treatment is ineffective over time.

When symptoms from two or three meridians simultaneously appear, it is referred to as combined diseases. If symptoms from one meridian persist, and symptoms from another meridian appear subsequently, it is termed concurrent diseases. For example, epigastric pain may be accompanied by heavy bleeding, abdominal pain, syncope, and nausea.

If pathogenic factors are not completely expelled, the righteous qi remains weakened, or new pathogenic factors are encountered, or if there is excessive exertion, dietary indiscretions, or improper use of medications, it may damage the righteous qi and assist the pathogenic factors, leading to a relapse.

**Weak and Strong Pathogenic Qi**

Let's discuss the issue of the waxing and waning of pathogenic and righteous qi.

Even when pathogenic qi is strong, as long as the righteous qi is not severely compromised, it can rise to combat the pathogenic factors. The outcome of the intense struggle between pathogenic and righteous qi is often manifested in the form of excess heat syndromes. Conditions arising from the stagnation of phlegm, food, water, blood, etc., such as the accumulation of phlegm and saliva, undigested food, excessive water and dampness, or stasis of blood, are all considered excess syndromes.

Deficiency syndromes are characterized by the specific manifestations of the decline in organ functions and are generally more common in the later stages and chronic processes of diseases. Conditions such as severe or prolonged illnesses that consume essence and qi, or conditions involving significant sweating, vomiting, diarrhea, or profuse bleeding that deplete the body's qi, blood, and fluids, can lead to a weakening of righteous qi, resulting in symptoms of deficiency of yin, yang, qi, and blood.

Throughout the course of a disease, the fluctuation and interplay of pathogenic and righteous qi often lead to complex pathological changes, including patterns where deficiency coexists with excess, excess coexists with deficiency, true and false deficiencies and excesses, and the mutual transformation of deficiencies and excesses.

**Imbalanced Yin and Yang**

During the course of a disease, due to the effects of pathogenic factors, the body's balance of yin and yang is lost, resulting in pathological changes where yin does not restrain yang and yang does not restrain yin.

The waxing and waning of yin and yang refer to the relative excess or deficiency of yin and yang, manifesting as either cold or hot, and either excess or deficiency pathological changes. The manifestations include four types: excess yang, excess yin, deficiency of yang, and deficiency of yin.

For example, in the initial stages of a common cold, symptoms such as severe chills with slight fever, headache and body aches, joint pain, nasal congestion with discharge, absence of sweating, cough, a thin white tongue coating, and a floating tight pulse may appear, indicating a yin pattern. If treated incorrectly, or due to constitutional factors, it may progress to symptoms of excess yang heat, such as high fever, sweating, irritability, thirst, a red tongue, a yellow coating, and a rapid pulse.

### Imbalanced Qi and Blood

Similar to the waxing and waning of pathogenic and righteous qi and the imbalance of yin and yang, the imbalance of qi and blood is not only the basis for various pathological changes in organs, meridians, and other aspects but also forms the foundation for analyzing and studying the pathogenesis of various diseases.

When qi is in motion, blood circulates; when qi stagnates, blood stasis occurs. Qi guides the flow of water, and when qi stagnates, water retention occurs. Therefore, qi stagnation can lead to blood stasis, water retention, and the development of pathological changes such as blood stasis, phlegm-dampness, and edema.

Abnormalities in the circulation of qi, as well as the decline in the physiological functions of qi, manifest specifically as qi deficiency, qi sinking, qi stagnation, reversed qi flow, qi blockage, and qi escaping.

Irregularities in the circulation of blood and a decline in blood's nourishing function include conditions like blood deficiency, blood stasis, blood heat, and bleeding.

When the relationship between qi and blood is disrupted, it primarily involves aspects such as qi stagnation leading to blood stasis, qi failing to control blood, qi escaping with blood, deficiency of both qi and blood, and inadequate nourishment of the meridians by qi and blood.

### Abnormal Distribution of Bodily Fluids

The abnormal distribution of bodily fluids and the imbalance between the generation and excretion of fluids lead to insufficient production, irregular distribution, or hindrances in excretion of bodily fluids. As a result, the circulation of bodily fluids within the body becomes sluggish, causing the accumulation of dampness, primarily giving rise to pathological changes such as obstruction by damp turbidity, condensation of phlegm-dampness, and retention of water.

The imbalance in the relationship between bodily fluids and qi and blood commonly manifests clinically as obstruction by water with qi stagnation, loss of qi with fluid discharge, depletion of bodily fluids leading to blood dryness, and deficiency of bodily fluids causing blood stasis.

### Five Internal Pathogenic Factors

In the process of disease development, pathological changes occur due to the abnormal functions of qi, blood, bodily fluids, and organs, resembling the pathogenic influences of the Six Exogenous Evils: wind, cold, summer heat, dampness, dryness, and fire. Since the origin of the disease is internal, these are respectively referred to as internal wind, internal cold, internal dampness, internal dryness, and internal fire, collectively known as the Five Internal Pathogenic Factors.

### Internal Wind Movement

The internal movement of wind qi is divided into excess and deficiency types, mainly including extreme heat generating wind, liver yang transforming into wind, yin deficiency generating wind movement, and blood deficiency generating wind.

Excessive heat generating wind movement is often seen in the critical phase of heat diseases. Due to the excessive pathogenic heat scorching the body fluids and damaging the nutritive blood, burning the liver meridian, this leads to the tendons and vessels losing their nourishment. Clinically, this is characterized by high fever, delirium, convulsions, rigidity, opisthotonos, upward staring of the eyes, etc.

Liver yang transforming into wind often results from emotional stress, overexertion depleting the yin of the liver and kidney, leading to yin deficiency and yang hyperactivity. Clinically, this can be seen as twitching muscles, numbness and trembling of limbs, dizziness and a tendency to fall, deviation of the mouth and eyes, hemiplegia, or sudden collapse due to blood following the reverse flow of qi, leading to syncope or collapse.

Yin deficiency generating wind movement; often seen in the late stage of heat diseases, due to the depletion of yin fluids or from long-term illness consuming the yin fluids. Clinically, this can be observed as muscle cramps and twitching, involuntary movements of hands and feet, and signs of yin fluid deficiency.

Blood deficiency, either due to insufficient blood production, excessive blood loss, or long-term illness depleting the nutritive blood, leads to insufficient liver blood, causing the tendons and vessels to lose nourishment, or the blood not nourishing the channels. Clinically, this can present as numbness of limbs, muscle twitches, extremities' contracture, and signs of yin and blood deficiency.

**Internal Cold**

Internal cold often arises due to deficiency of yang qi, leading to an excess of yin-cold within the body when the warming function is impaired. When warmth is deficient, internal cold emerges, presenting symptoms of insufficient yang heat, such as pale complexion and cold limbs.

In cases where cold nature causes stagnation, its contracting quality leads to the contraction of tendons and vessels, causing sluggish blood circulation, resulting in muscle spasms and pain in the limbs. When yang qi is deficient, the functions of qi transformation and control are impaired, preventing the warming and transformation of fluids. This can lead to the accumulation or stagnation of pathogenic products related to yin-cold, such as water, dampness, and phlegm. Consequently, excretions like urine, phlegm, mucus, and saliva appear clear and cold, or there may be symptoms such as diarrhea or edema.

**Internal Dampness**

The generation of internal dampness is often associated with factors such as obesity and excessive accumulation of phlegm-dampness. Additionally, it can result from indulging in raw and cold foods, overconsumption of fatty and sweet foods, and internal damage to the spleen and stomach, leading to impaired transportation of fluids and hindrance in the distribution of bodily fluids.

The key to the internal generation of dampness lies in the malfunction of the spleen's transforming function. Dampness is characterized by a heavy, sticky, and sluggish nature, primarily obstructing the middle burner involving the spleen and stomach. This manifests as distension and fullness in the epigastric and abdominal regions, poor appetite, a sticky or sweet taste in the mouth, and a thick, greasy tongue coating. If dampness stagnates in the lower burner, symptoms may include abdominal distension, loose stools, and difficulty in urination. When water and dampness overflow into the skin and muscles, it can lead to edema. If dampness affects the upper burner, symptoms such as chest tightness, coughing, and wheezing may occur.

**Internal Dryness**

In cases of internal dryness, manifestations include dry cough and dryness in the throat and mouth in the upper burner; restlessness, thirst, and hiccups in the middle burner; and constipation and menstrual blockage in the lower burner. Clinically, it is often associated with the pattern of yin deficiency and internal heat due to the depletion of bodily fluids.

Symptoms of internal dryness may include dry and non-moisturized skin, peeling or cracking, severe cases may lead to fissures. Other signs include dry mouth, parched throat, and cracked lips. The tongue may lack moisture and could be excessively red with cracks, and the nose and eyes may also feel dry and gritty. Bowel movements may be dry and difficult, and urine may be short and red, indicating a dry-heat pattern.

If lung dryness is predominant, additional symptoms may include a dry cough without phlegm, and in severe cases, there may be coughing up of blood. When stomach dryness is predominant, there may be insufficient stomach yin, and the tongue may appear red and shiny. If kidney dryness is predominant, it indicates depletion of kidney yin, leading to symptoms such as body thinning, hair loss, premature graying, and in severe cases, menstrual blockage and wilting. In cases of intestinal dryness, symptoms may include constipation.

**Internal Heat**

The pathological manifestations of internal heat and fire can be broadly categorized into excess and deficiency. Excessive fire often originates from an excess of yang qi, the transformation of stagnated pathogenic factors into fire, or the transformation of the Five Emotions into fire. The progression of this condition is rapid, with a relatively short course, and is characterized by strong fever, flushed face, preference for cold drinks, yellow-red urine, constipation, and in severe cases, agitation, delirium, a dry and yellow tongue coating, and a rapid, forceful pulse.

Deficient fire is often attributed to insufficient essence and blood, where yin deficiency fails to restrain yang, leading to an upsurge of deficient yang. The progression of this condition is slow, with a longer course. Clinical features include a persistent sensation of heat in the five centers (heart, hands, feet, chest, and abdomen), afternoon flushing of the cheeks, insomnia with night sweats, dry mouth, and throat, dizziness, tinnitus, a red tongue with scanty coating, and a thin, rapid pulse.

## Pathology of the Zang-fu Organs

The heart governs the blood vessels and houses the spirit. Its radiance manifests on the face, its sensory opening is the tongue, and it corresponds to the Hand Shaoyin meridian. Additionally, it is interconnected with the Small Intestine on both a superficial and deep level. These specific connections in function constitute the cardiovascular system. Therefore, pathological changes in the heart reflect abnormal reactions at various levels of this system, mainly evident in the aspects of blood vessels and the spirit.

Regarding blood vessels, cold causes blood stasis, leading to chest pain and cold extremities. Heat causes excessive blood circulation, resulting in a red complexion and bleeding. Deficiency leads to weak circulation, poor blood flow, a weak or hesitant pulse. Excess causes poor circulation, blood vessel obstruction, stagnant blood flow, and the harm of blood stasis.

Concerning the spirit, cold leads to insufficient spirit, resulting in a calm demeanor and a desire to curl up and sleep. In severe cases, excessive cold may lead to an abrupt loss of yang, resulting in unclear consciousness. Heat causes the spirit to lose control, leading to restlessness, agitation, insomnia, and even delirium. Deficiency results in fatigue, sluggish speech, and a lack of vitality. Excess manifests as unpredictable mood swings, overwhelming sadness, or even mania. Sweat is considered the fluid of the heart. After profuse sweating, if the heart yang is depleted, it can lead to flaming up of heart fire, causing a red and painful tongue. If the heart fire descends to the Small Intestine, it may result in painful and difficult urination with red urine.

The pathological changes in the lungs primarily manifest as abnormal respiratory function, imbalances in fluid metabolism, dysfunction of the body surface barrier, as well as disturbances in the generation of Qi, circulatory disorders, and certain skin conditions.

Pathological changes in the lungs can be categorized into Excess and Deficiency. Excess conditions may include heat accumulation, phlegm obstruction, water accumulation, or blood stasis. Deficiency conditions may involve Qi deficiency, Yin deficiency, or a deficiency in both Qi and Yin. Deficiency conditions in the lungs often arise from the transformation of Excess conditions, and there can be a complex interplay between excess and deficiency.

The spleen, as the Tai Yin Earth organ, relies on its Yang Qi for proper function. Dysfunction in the transforming function of the spleen primarily results from a deficiency in its Yang Qi, leading to an inability to ascend and clarify. The role of the spleen in controlling blood circulation is essentially the manifestation of the stabilizing effect of its Yang Qi. Therefore, pathological changes in the spleen mainly revolve around the imbalance of its Yang Qi.

In spleen diseases, Qi deficiency is the foundation, and dampness is the manifestation. The spleen governs the transformation of water and dampness, so spleen deficiency leads to the stagnation of water and dampness, hindering its transformation. This, in turn, affects the spleen's overall function. Spleen deficiency with dampness is a pathological change where spleen deficiency leads to internal dampness obstruction. Clinical characteristics include signs of spleen Qi deficiency, along with symptoms such as epigastric and abdominal fullness and pain, fatigue in the limbs, reduced appetite, a bland or sticky taste in the mouth, nausea, loose stools, and in severe cases, edema and a white, greasy tongue coating.

Qi, fire, and wind are significant characteristics in the pathological development process of the liver. Liver Qi stagnation is the manifestation of the liver's failure to disperse and move Qi, leading to Qi stagnation and blockage. When the liver's Qi is stagnant and not flowing smoothly, it can transform into liver fire. Prolonged liver fire can consume liver Yin, leading to an imbalance with liver Yang, resulting in liver Yang ascending excessively.

When liver Yang is uncontrolled and rises, leading to internal movement of wind, it manifests as liver wind (transformation of liver Yang into wind). Among these factors, liver Qi stagnation is often the primary cause, serving as the initiating factor for liver diseases. Additionally, in the pathological progression involving Qi and blood, Qi stagnation can lead to blood stasis, and when Qi stagnation is prolonged, it may result in phlegm accumulation due to blocked fluid circulation. The pathological changes involving Qi, fire, phlegm, blood stasis, and wind can give rise to various complex diseases, and their pathological roots are often related to liver Qi stagnation.

The pathological changes in the kidneys are characterized by deficiency rather than excess, with manifestations of both cold and heat imbalances. Kidney deficiency can be classified into two main types: Yin deficiency and Yang deficiency.

Kidney Yang deficiency involves a depletion of the warming function, resulting in insufficient life-gate fire and weakened kidney Qi, leading to pathological changes such as overall physiological decline, impaired fluid metabolism, disturbances in the spleen and stomach's transformation of water and grains, diminished reproductive function, and dysfunction in the ascending and descending of lung Qi.

Kidney Qi instability often occurs due to age-related weakness in kidney Qi, insufficient kidney Qi in the young, or prolonged illness depleting kidney Qi. This results in an inability of the kidney Qi to stabilize and contain, leading to clinical symptoms such as nocturnal emissions, spermatorrhea, premature ejaculation, urinary incontinence, dribbling after urination, enuresis, irregular or continuous menstruation, excessive menstruation, vaginal discharge, miscarriage, and chronic diarrhea due to weakened bowel control.

Kidney inability to receive Qi is frequently observed in patients with a prolonged history of coughing and wheezing, often preceded by lung Qi deficiency. Over time, this condition affects the kidneys, leading to a comprehensive presentation of kidney Qi deficiency. Clinical manifestations include a combination of excess above and deficiency below, difficulty breathing, increased breathlessness with exertion, and an imbalance in inhalation and exhalation.

In pathological terms, the gallbladder often manifests as excess Yang and excessive heat, with predominance of tangible symptoms. The presence of heat can scorch bodily fluids and lead to the formation of phlegm, resulting in gallbladder disorders commonly accompanied by the presence of phlegm. Phlegm and stagnant heat obstructing the gallbladder can easily disturb the mind and spirit.

The stomach's functional imbalances primarily manifest as abnormalities in its receiving and ripening functions, as well as stomach Qi rebelliously ascending due to a loss of harmony between the ascending and descending functions.

Pathological changes in the small intestine are mainly reflected in abnormal bowel movements. Major clinical presentations include difficult urination, diarrhea as the main symptom, bloating and indigestion due to failure in digesting food, and vomiting and abdominal pain with intestinal rumbling caused by the failure to separate clear from turbid substances. Small intestine excess heat is often attributed to the downward influx of damp heat or the transfer of heart heat to the small intestine, leading to frequent urination or cloudy urine. Small intestine deficiency cold is mostly related to dietary irregularities and damage to the spleen and stomach, resulting in symptoms such as intestinal rumbling, diarrhea, and abdominal pain that worsens with pressure.

The pathological mechanisms of the large intestine mainly manifest as functional disorders leading to abnormal bowel movements. Excessive heat accumulation in the large intestine is often caused by internal dryness and heat congestion, the transfer of lung heat to the large intestine, or the accumulation of damp-heat, resulting in a lack of moisture in the large intestine and constipation. If damp-heat accumulates in the large intestine or if cold-damp transforms into heat, it may lead to diarrhea. If damp-heat conflicts with Qi and blood, symptoms such as red or white dysentery, urgency with difficulty in completing bowel movements may occur. When damp-heat obstructs meridians, Qi stagnates, and blood stasis occurs, it can lead to the formation of hemorrhoids and anal fistulas.

Large intestine deficiency cold, characterized by a decline in Spleen Yang and abnormal digestion function, or kidney Yang deficiency leading to internal accumulation of Yin and cold, can result in loose stools, failure to digest grains properly, and even incontinence.

The bladder's gasification function relies on the gasification role of the kidneys. If the kidneys fail to contain and store, gasification loses its authority, leading to symptoms like enuresis and urinary incontinence. Bladder deficiency cold is often due to kidney Qi deficiency, lack of containment, and loss of bladder control, resulting in frequent, clear, or involuntary urination, dribbling after urination, and weak urination.

### Pathology by Differentiating the Meridians

The twelve meridians have specific connections with the five Zang organs and six Fu organs. Therefore, when the twelve meridians are affected, it can influence the corresponding Zang-Fu organs, leading to pathological changes in the organs.

If there is a deficiency of Qi and blood in the meridians, it can cause a decline in the physiological functions of the corresponding Zang-Fu organs, leading to the manifestation of diseases. For example, pathological changes in the Stomach Meridian of Foot Yangming can result in symptoms such as body heat, good appetite but frequent hunger, yellow and red urine, and even mania when the meridian Qi is excessive. Conversely, when the meridian Qi is deficient, symptoms like chills, spasms, abdominal bloating, and weakness or atrophy of the leg may occur.

When the Qi and blood circulation in the meridians is not smooth, it is due to the obstruction of meridian Qi, affecting the circulation of Qi and blood, often impacting the physiological functions of the Zang-Fu organs and the areas where the meridians pass through. For example, symptoms such as generalized muscle soreness and pain can be caused by the obstruction of superficial meridian Qi due to external pathogenic factors. The impaired circulation of Qi in the Liver Meridian of Foot Jueyin is a major cause of conditions like rib pain, nodules, lump in the throat, and breast lumps.

The hindrance of Qi in the meridians and the impaired circulation of Qi and blood in the meridians are major factors contributing to Qi stagnation and blood stasis in a particular meridian.

The Eight Extraordinary Meridians (Qi Jing Ba Mai) are interconnected with the twelve regular meridians and play a role in regulating the Qi and blood of the twelve main meridians. The Conception Vessel (Ren Mai) is related to gynecological and pregnancy-related conditions such as leaking amniotic fluid, threatened miscarriage, and abnormal vaginal discharge. As the vessel that binds and supports the fetus, weakness in the Conception Vessel may lead to difficulties in supporting the fetus, resulting in an unstable pregnancy. Conditions like weakness in the Conception Vessel may contribute to an increased risk of miscarriage, and injuries to the Conception Vessel can lead to an unstable pregnancy or abnormal vaginal discharge.

Diseases in one meridian are likely to affect other meridians connected to it, or influence other associated meridians. For instance, the Liver Meridian of Foot Jueyin travels through the hypochondriac region and connects to the Lungs. If there is Qi stagnation and constraint in the Liver, leading to the transformation of Qi into heat, Liver Fire may ascend along the meridian, injuring the Lung Meridian of Hand Taiyin. This interaction is referred to as the relationship of wood (Liver) generating fire (Heat) and fire (Heat) overcoming metal

(Lungs), resulting in symptoms such as chest and hypochondriac pain, coughing with blood-streaked sputum, and pain in the chest when coughing – reflecting the combined pathology of the Liver and Lung meridians.

The human body is an organic whole, and there are interconnected pathways between the surface and interior, as well as between the Zang-Fu organs. Therefore, a pathological condition in one area can extend and affect other areas, leading to the occurrence of diseases in those affected areas.

The Zang and Fu organs are mutually related in terms of interior-exterior connections, with changes occurring either from Zang to Fu or from Fu to Zang. Generally, diseases originating from Fu and affecting Zang are considered more severe, and Zang diseases are challenging to treat. Conversely, diseases originating from Zang and affecting Fu are considered less severe, and Fu diseases are more easily treatable.

The imbalance of Yin and Yang is the fundamental contradiction in diseases. Various diseases, in terms of the relationship between pathogenic and healthy factors, involve struggles, changes, and fluctuations in the balance between these factors. Therefore, in treatment, the fundamental principle is to support the healthy and expel the pathogenic.

Addressing the immediate symptoms when urgent and addressing the root causes when there is time are both crucial in treatment. When treating diseases, it is necessary to identify the fundamental causes, grasp the essence of the disease, and tailor treatment to address these root causes. This principle is a fundamental guideline in the traditional Chinese medicine approach to diagnosis and treatment.

The recovery and speed of recovery from a disease depend not only on the general health and resistance of the patient but also on timely, correct, and proactive treatment. Timely intervention and appropriate treatment play a crucial role in determining whether a disease can be cured and the speed of recovery.

# Chapter 7

# Basic Principles in Treatment

In traditional Chinese medicine, the general principles for treating diseases can be summarized as follows: address the root cause of the illness, strive for balance, understand the regular patterns and adapt to changes, and guide treatment based on the prevailing conditions.

The concepts of supporting the body's vital energy and dispelling pathogenic factors are interconnected aspects of TCM treatment. Supporting the body's vital energy aims to expel pathogenic factors by strengthening the body's inherent resilience. On the other hand, dispelling pathogenic factors is undertaken to support the body's vital energy by eliminating factors that contribute to illness, ultimately promoting the restoration of health.

Specific methods are as follows:

(1) Supporting the Body's Vital Energy: This approach is suitable for conditions where the primary imbalance is deficiency in the body's vital energy, and pathogenic factors are not excessively strong. For instance, when dealing with conditions such as qi deficiency or yang deficiency, it is advisable to employ methods that tonify qi and strengthen yang. In cases of yin deficiency or blood deficiency, treatments focusing on nourishing yin and replenishing blood are appropriate.

(2) Dispelling Pathogenic Factors: This method is applicable when the predominant imbalance is excess pathogenic factors, while the body's vital energy remains relatively strong. Clinical interventions

commonly include sweating therapy, vomiting therapy, purgation, clearing heat, promoting diuresis, resolving dampness, promoting qi circulation, and activating blood circulation. These approaches are developed based on the specific nature of the pathogenic factors present, guided by the principle of dispelling pathogenic factors.

(3) Attack before Tonifying: This means addressing pathogenic factors before supporting the body's vital energy. It is applicable when pathogenic factors are predominant and the body's vital energy is deficient but still resilient to attack. The main contradiction lies in the excess of pathogenic factors, and if tonifying is considered simultaneously, it may inadvertently assist the pathogenic factors. For example, in cases of excessive bleeding due to blood stasis, where blood stagnation needs to be resolved first to stop the bleeding before replenishing the blood.

(4) Tonify before Attacking: This approach involves supporting the body's vital energy before dispelling pathogenic factors. It is suitable for situations where there is a complex mix of deficiency and excess, and the body's vital energy is too weak to withstand immediate attack. In such cases, attacking pathogenic factors prematurely can further harm the body's vital energy. For instance, in conditions like abdominal distension where the primary contradiction is weakened vital energy, tonifying methods are employed first. Once the vital energy is sufficiently restored, then pathogenic factors can be addressed without causing unexpected complications.

(5) Combined Attack and Tonify: This approach involves simultaneously supporting the body's vital energy and dispelling pathogenic factors. It is suitable for cases where both deficiency and excess are present but not overly severe. The specific application requires distinguishing the primary and secondary aspects of deficiency and excess, using a flexible approach. For example, when deficiency is the main contradiction, and solely tonifying might allow pathogenic factors to linger, a combined approach of tonifying and dispelling is

appropriate. In the case of a Qi-deficient cold, the emphasis should be on tonifying Qi while simultaneously resolving the exterior. Conversely, when excess pathogenic factors are the main issue, and attacking alone might harm the body's vital energy, the primary focus should be on dispelling pathogenic factors while supporting the body's vital energy.

**Treating Both the Root Causes and Symptoms**

The theory of "root and branch" holds significant guiding significance for accurately analyzing the illness, distinguishing the primary and secondary factors, understanding the essential and non-essential aspects, and assessing the severity and urgency of the disease, leading to the application of appropriate treatment.

The application of the theory of "Root and Branch" in treatment:

(1) Treating the Root in a Gradual Manner: This principle is generally applicable to chronic diseases or instances where the disease tends to improve, the body's vital energy is weakened, and pathogenic factors have not yet been fully expelled. For example, in the case of internally generated illnesses that progress gradually, and when the qi and blood of the organs have already declined, treatment should wait until the essential qi of the organs is sufficient for the body's vital energy to gradually recover.

(2) Addressing the Manifestations in Urgent Cases: This principle is generally applicable to acute and severe conditions, or when certain symptoms pose a life-threatening risk during the course of the disease. For instance, in the treatment of sudden and severe illnesses, it is not advisable to delay treatment. When the pathogenic factors are not deeply entrenched in the early stages of the disease, prompt treatment is essential to expel the pathogenic factors without harming the body's vital energy, facilitating a faster recovery for the patient.

**Method of Simultaneous Treatment**

Treating Both the Root and Branch refers to simultaneously addressing both the root cause and the manifestations. This approach is applicable when both the primary and secondary aspects of the disease are urgent. For example, in the case of a patient with dysentery, the inability to eat is a sign of weakened vital energy (root), while persistent diarrhea indicates an excess of pathogenic factors (manifestation). In such situations where both aspects are urgent, a combination of tonifying the body's vital energy and clearing damp-heat remedies is necessary. This approach is an example of the method of simultaneous treatment.

Another example is a patient with spleen deficiency and qi stagnation. Spleen deficiency is the root cause, and qi stagnation is the manifestation. To address the root cause, herbs like ginseng, white atractylodes, poria, and licorice are used to tonify the spleen and supplement qi. Simultaneously, herbs like muxiang, sha ren, and chenpi are added to regulate qi and resolve stagnation, addressing the manifestation. This dual treatment strategy is another example.

**Direct Treatment and Contrary Treatment**

Direct treatment is the most commonly used therapeutic principle in clinical practice. This principle involves treating conditions by counteracting the nature of the symptoms. Since diseases can be categorized by characteristics such as cold, heat, deficiency, and excess, the direct treatment method involves warming the cold, cooling the heat, tonifying the deficiency, and purging the excess.

Contrary treatment, on the other hand, is a therapeutic principle that involves treating diseases by following the false appearances of the disease.

This involves using warm-natured medicinal substances to treat diseases that exhibit false heat symptoms. It is suitable for true cold false heat syndromes, where yin cold is abundant internally, obstructing yang on the outside, resulting in a situation where there is true cold inside and false heat outside. During treatment, the essence of the disease is addressed by using warm-natured medicines to treat the true cold. Once the true cold is eliminated, the false heat will also disappear.

Using cold-natured medicinal substances to treat diseases exhibiting false cold symptoms is a therapeutic method. This is suitable for true heat false cold syndromes where there is excessive internal heat, and the dominance of yang suppresses yin. For example, in the case of heat collapse syndrome, where internal yang is excessive, suppressing yin externally, only false cold symptoms such as cold limbs are evident. However, the essence of the disease lies in symptoms like strong fever, thirst, dry stools, and dark urine. Therefore, using cold remedies to address the true heat will naturally eliminate the false cold.

Using tonifying medicines to treat diseases with symptoms of blockage or obstruction is a therapeutic method. This is applicable to true deficiency false excess syndromes caused by deficiency leading to blockage or obstruction. For instance, in cases of abdominal distension due to weak spleen and stomach, where the Qi mechanism is disrupted, tonifying the spleen and supplementing the stomach is necessary to restore the proper function of the spleen and stomach, allowing the Qi mechanism to function normally and relieving the abdominal distension.

Using promoting and regulating medicines to treat diseases with symptoms of excess and stagnation is a therapeutic method. This is suitable for syndromes with a combination of true excess and false deficiency, such as treating food stagnation with diarrhea by using methods of promoting digestion and regulating bowel movements, or treating irregular menstruation caused by blood stasis with methods that promote blood circulation and resolve stasis. This approach involves using promoting and regulating methods to address both excess and deficiency aspects.

**Regulating the Yin and Yang**

The concept of adjusting Yin and Yang involves addressing imbalances in the relative excess or deficiency of Yin and Yang within the body. It follows the principle of reducing the excessive and supplementing the deficient to restore Yin and Yang to a relatively balanced state.

Therapeutic methods such as releasing exterior conditions, attacking interior conditions, promoting clarity while descending turbidity, tonifying deficiencies and purging excesses, and regulating Qi and blood all fall within the scope of adjusting Yin and Yang. These approaches aim to restore a relative balance between Yin and Yang by addressing imbalances in the body's energetic forces.

**Harmonizing Qi and Blood**

The concept of harmonizing Qi and blood involves addressing deficiencies and abnormalities in the functions of Qi and blood. If there is an excess, it is purged, and if there is a deficiency, it is supplemented, ultimately aiming to promote the smooth flow and harmony of Qi and blood.

In the treatment of Qi-related conditions, in summary, tonification is applied for Qi deficiency, dispersion for Qi stagnation, lifting for Qi sinking, lowering for Qi rebellion, stabilizing for Qi escaping, and opening for Qi obstruction.

Qi-tonifying medicines are prone to causing stagnation. Generally, in cases of internal phlegm-damp accumulation, their use is not advisable. However, when necessary, combining Qi tonification with phlegm-transforming and dampness-expelling methods may be considered.

Qi-dispersing medicines are often pungent and drying. Large doses or prolonged use can deplete Qi, disperse Qi excessively, and consume body fluids. Caution is needed when using these medicines for conditions involving blood deficiency, Yin deficiency, or excessive internal heat.

In clinical practice, blood-related disorders include blood deficiency, blood stasis, bleeding, cold blood, and hot blood. Their treatments involve nourishing blood, promoting blood circulation, stopping bleeding, and cooling blood, each addressing specific aspects of the condition.

Blood deficiency and Yin deficiency are often interrelated, so for cases of blood deficiency accompanied by Yin deficiency, complementary herbs to nourish Yin are commonly combined to enhance their effects. Blood-nourishing medicines are often rich and greasy, which can hinder digestion. Therefore, caution is advised when using them for conditions involving dampness accumulation in the middle Jiao, abdominal distension, and reduced appetite with loose stools.

Although promoting blood circulation and resolving blood stasis is a general principle for treating blood stasis conditions, the severity and urgency of blood stasis may vary. Accordingly, treatment methods such as harmonizing blood and promoting blood circulation, activating blood and resolving blood stasis, and breaking blood and expelling blood stasis should be employed in sequence, starting with milder methods before progressing to more intense ones. It is crucial not to overlook the severity of blood stasis and use overly aggressive measures, as this may result in the removal of blood stasis at the expense of harming the body.

"Treating cold with warmth and treating warmth with cold" is a fundamental principle in traditional Chinese medicine. Blood stasis may have either a cold or hot nature. Therefore, the selection of medications should consider their thermal properties, choosing them based on whether they are cold, hot, warm, or cool.

In clinical practice, blood-related disorders present various patterns, including blood deficiency, blood stasis, bleeding, cold in the blood, and heat in the blood. The treatment approaches for these conditions differ, involving methods such as nourishing blood, promoting blood circulation, stopping bleeding, and cooling the blood.

Blood deficiency and Yin deficiency often interact as cause and effect. Therefore, when treating blood deficiency coexisting with Yin deficiency, it is common to combine herbs that tonify Yin to enhance their effects. Blood-tonifying herbs are often rich and nourishing, which may hinder digestion. Hence, caution is advised when using them for conditions involving damp stagnation in the middle burner, abdominal distension, and loose stools.

Although promoting blood circulation and resolving blood stasis is a general principle for treating blood stasis, the severity and urgency of blood stasis should be considered. Depending on the degree of blood stasis, a sequential approach may be adopted, involving methods like harmonizing blood circulation, promoting blood circulation and resolving blood stasis, and breaking blood to expel stasis. It is crucial not to indiscriminately break up blood stasis without considering its severity, as it may harm the body's normal functions once the stasis is removed.

The principle of "treating cold with heat and treating heat with cold" is a fundamental concept in traditional Chinese medicine. For blood stasis, the underlying causes may be related to cold or heat. Therefore, the choice of herbal medicine should be based on their temperature properties (cold, hot, warm, cool).

Certain blood-activating and stasis-resolving herbs are particularly sensitive to specific diseases or affected areas. For example, San Leng, E Zhu, and Wei Ling Xian are used to disperse masses and eliminate obstruction. Huang Yao Zi and Liu Ji Nu are used for treating lumps. Chuan Xiong is used for blood stasis in the upper body, while Niu Xi is used for the lower body. Yu Jin is used for blood stasis in the heart, and Ze Lan is used for the liver. Understanding the nature of these herbs helps in creating precise and effective herbal formulations.

Blood tends to coagulate when it gets cold and flow smoothly when it gets warm. Therefore, the use of cooling blood and stopping bleeding herbs, as well as clearing heat and cooling blood herbs, should be done cautiously to avoid excessive dosages. When there is evident stasis in bleeding, it is not advisable to use large doses of cold herbs to stop bleeding alone. In such cases, combining herbs that promote blood circulation is necessary to prevent the retention of stasis.

In the early stages of blood disorders, large doses of cooling and blood-stopping herbs should be avoided, and cold herbs should not be used for an extended period to prevent blood stasis and damage to the spleen yang. It is crucial to refrain from solely using astringent and blood-stopping herbs, as this may lead to retaining the pathogenic factors. The use of charcoalized herbs as a hemostatic agent is an essential measure in traditional Chinese medicine. However, it should not be used indiscriminately for all bleeding cases without considering the nature of the disease, deficiency or excess conditions, and the temperature properties of the herbs.

For bleeding due to deficiency heat and excessive fire, it is advisable to nourish Yin, clear heat, and reduce fire. The use of sweet and cold or salty and cold herbs is suitable for nourishing Yin, clearing heat, and reducing fire. Charcoal preparations, with their scorching and bitter properties, have the potential to damage body fluids and consume liquids, so they are not recommended in this context. If there is a combination of deficiency and excess, with bleeding occurring, it is appropriate to consider both cold and hot properties in the herbs. Whether the hemostatic agent is cold or hot, charcoalized herbs can be used.

Qi deficiency inevitably leads to blood deficiency, weakened propulsion, and warming functions that can lead to blood stasis. If the function of governing and controlling is weakened, it can result in bleeding. Qi stagnation can lead to blood stasis, and if the Qi mechanism is disrupted, blood can move abnormally, either rising or sinking.

Blood follows the movement of Qi, and when Qi is harmonious, blood circulates along the meridians. If Qi rebels, blood may overflow chaotically. In cases of liver stagnation and Qi stagnation, where the dispersing and regulating functions are compromised, blood stasis may occur. Therefore, herbs that soothe the liver and regulate Qi are necessary to promote the smooth flow of Qi, and when Qi flows, so does the blood.

In summary, treating Qi without addressing blood is not a complete treatment. Treating blood requires addressing Qi. When the Qi mechanism is regulated, blood disorders can be cured.

**Personalized Treatment**

Adapt the treatment to the season, the location, and the individual.

Adhering to the principle of adapting treatment to the characteristics of different seasons involves considering the climatic features when determining the therapeutic approach. For instance, during the spring and summer seasons when the weather gradually warms, and the Yang Qi is ascending, the body's pores become more relaxed and open. Even if there is an external invasion of wind-cold, one should be cautious in using strong diaphoretic and dispersing herbs like ephedra and cinnamon, to avoid excessive sweating that might deplete Qi and Yin. In contrast, during the autumn and winter seasons when the climate becomes colder and the Yang Qi wanes, and the body's pores tighten, if there is a heat syndrome, one should also exercise caution in using cold herbs like gypsum and mint to prevent excessive coldness that may harm Yang.

Considering the geographical environment when determining the therapeutic approach is known as adapting to the location. For example, when treating an exterior wind-cold syndrome with herbs like ephedra and cinnamon, in extremely cold regions of the northwest, the dosage can be slightly heavier, whereas in the warm and hot southeast regions, the dosage should be lighter.

Adapting the treatment to the patient's age, gender, constitution, lifestyle, and other individual characteristics is referred to as personalized treatment.

In the case of elderly individuals, who often experience a decline in Qi and blood, reduced physical activities, and are prone to deficiency syndromes or a combination of deficiency and excess, the treatment approach should focus on tonifying deficiencies for those with deficiency syndromes. However, when dealing with a combination of deficiency and excess, especially when attacking pathogenic factors, careful consideration of herbal formulations is necessary to avoid compromising the body's vital energy.

Children have vigorous vitality, but their Qi and blood are relatively insufficient, and their organs are delicate. Additionally, infants and young children are unable to manage their own lives, often experiencing irregular feeding, imbalances in temperature, and susceptibility to illnesses. Therefore, when treating children, caution is advised against using strong purgatives and tonics.

For women, factors such as menstrual cycles, pregnancy, and postpartum conditions must be taken into account when prescribing medications. During pregnancy, the use of drastic purgatives, blood-breaking herbs, slippery and dispersing herbs, as well as toxic substances, should be avoided or used cautiously to prevent harm to the fetus. Postpartum considerations include addressing deficiencies in Qi and blood and monitoring lochia conditions.

The treatment principles of adapting to the season, location, and individual needs demonstrate the holistic perspective and the flexibility of the differential diagnosis and treatment approach in traditional Chinese medicine. It emphasizes the importance of considering various factors and tailoring the treatment plan to the specific circumstances of each patient.

As my dear readers, you can find more detailed discussions on each of the above topics in other TCM books written by me. Or you can reach me here: isherhope@gmail.com

Thank you.